Understanding Syndrome

Understanding Tourette Syndrome provides accessible, concise, evidence-based guidelines on this neurodevelopmental disorder, offering parents and professionals a deeper scientific understanding of the condition and its consequences. Zanaboni Dina and Porta explore signs, symptoms and treatment of the disease, with the aim of demonstrating to all those involved in the life of a TS child solutions to manage a range of situations from diagnosis to day-to-day life.

Therapies and social intervention, including Habit Reversal Training and Deep Brain Stimulation, are described, allowing caregivers to evaluate the best course of treatment. With a focus on improving quality of life by offering practical recommendations for managing the condition at school and in the family, it places additional emphasis on sibling relationships and the importance of childhood friendship. The authors' expert subject knowledge and extensive experience of working with children and families, makes the topic accessible for any reader, and case studies demonstrate how to apply scientific understanding of the condition to a real-life situation.

This unique guide is essential reading for parents and carers, as well as practitioners in Clinical and Educational Psychology, Counselling, Mental Health, Nursing, Child Welfare, Public Healthcare and those in Education. It will also be of interest to postgraduates studying courses in Psychology, Neurology and Psychiatry.

Carlotta Zanaboni Dina is psychologist and psychotherapist of AIST (Italian Association for TS patients), and trainer of two CBT Academies. She has been working at the Tourette Syndrome Centre, Milan, Italy, for 10 years. She previously conducted her studies at the Yale Child Study Center, US, with Professor Leckman, and also in London, UK, namely with Professor Robertson and Dr. Hedderly's team at Guy's and St. Thomas' Hospital.

Mauro Porta, neurologist, is former Teaching Professor of the University of Milan, founder of AIST, and Director of the Extrapyramidal Diseases and Tourette Syndrome Centre at Galeazzi Clinical and Research Hospital, Milan, Italy. He worked at the Northwestern University of Chicago, USA, and got a Master Degree in Functional Neurosurgery. Named also as "Charcot's son", Mauro spent several years working at the Salpêtrière Hospital of Paris, birthplace of Tourette syndrome.

Understanding Atypical Development

Series editor: Alessandro Antonietti, Università Cattolica del Sacro Cuore, Italy.

This volume is one of a rapidly developing series in *Understanding Atypical Development*, published by Routledge. This book series is a set of basic, concise guides on various developmental disorders or issues of atypical development. The books are aimed at parents, but also professionals in health, education, social care and related fields, and are focused on providing insights into the aspects of the condition that can be troubling to children, and what can be done about it. Each volume is grounded in scientific theory but with an accessible writing style, making them ideal for a wide variety of audiences.

Each volume in the series is published in hardback, paperback and eBook formats. More information about the series is available on the official website at: https://www.routledge.com/Understanding-Atypical-Development/book-series/UATYPDEV, including details of all the titles published to date.

Published Titles

Understanding Tourette Syndrome
By Carlotta Zanaboni Dina and Mauro Porta

Understanding Rett Syndrome
By Rosa Angela Fabio, Tindara Caprì and Gabriella Martino

Understanding Conduct Disorder and Oppositional-Defiant Disorder
Laura Vanzin & Valentina Mauri

Understanding Tourette Syndrome

A guide to symptoms, management and treatment

Edited by Carlotta Zanaboni Dina and Mauro Porta

Foreword by James F. Leckman

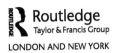

Routledge
Taylor & Francis Group

LONDON AND NEW YORK

First published 2020
by Routledge
2 Park Square, Milton Park, Abingdon, Oxon OX14 4RN

and by Routledge
52 Vanderbilt Avenue, New York, NY 10017

Routledge is an imprint of the Taylor & Francis Group, an informa business

British Library Cataloguing-in-Publication Data
A catalogue record for this book is available from the British Library

Library of Congress Cataloging-in-Publication Data
A catalog record has been requested for this book

ISBN: 978-1-138-59559-0 (hbk)
ISBN: 978-1-138-59560-6 (pbk)
ISBN: 978-0-429-48820-7 (ebk)

Typeset in Sabon
by Swales & Willis Ltd, Exeter, Devon, UK

To understand a child's needs, kneel down
and listen.

Contents

Foreword

by Professor James F. Leckman

Carlotta Zanaboni Dina and Mauro Porta have done a superb job in presenting a detailed and up-to-date guide to understanding the complexities of Tourette syndrome. Tourette is an enigmatic condition. Its etiology includes a multiplicity of both genetic and environmental factors. Likewise, its symptomatic presentation and clinical course varies from individual to individual. It typically includes not only motor and "sound" tics but also, to a lesser or greater degree, a broad spectrum of other symptoms including attentional difficulties; intrusive, repetitive ideas (obsessions) and repetitive undesired actions (compulsions); as well as impulsive behaviors. A minority of individuals also present with difficulties in social-emotional reciprocity and social communication that fall on the autism spectrum.

While more research is needed to optimize and personalize the available treatment options, Carlotta Zanaboni Dina and Mauro Porta have expertly summarized the current treatments of proven value. They range from cognitive-behavioral approaches to use of pharmaceutical agents and neuromodulatory procedures. In addition to providing guidance to clinicians how best to proceed with regard to treatment, they also reflect on the importance of the individual's microbiota as well as immunomodulatory and dietary interventions.

Importantly, this volume also conveys to clinicians that they must not lose sight of the individual's family, school and social networks as they engage and care for children, adolescents and adults with Tourette syndrome. They encourage clinicians to consider the vast complexity of the individual's life from biological, psychological, and social perspectives and the need to build on the individual's strengths and to keep their development and life trajectories on track. Their approach is well illustrated in the final chapter where

"Giuseppe's" life journey in dealing with his tics and obsessive-compulsive symptoms is presented in detail. Over the course of more than a decade of therapeutic engagement, he responded well to a range of interventions that involved not only Giuseppe, but also his family and school personnel.

In addition to being an invaluable guide to clinicians and practitioners, the content of *Understanding Tourette Syndrome* is presented in such a way that it is immediately accessible, through creative illustrations and photographs, to patients and their families as well as to teachers and others who have an interest in learning more about this syndrome. Indeed, the very first chapter of this volume is devoted to presenting its historical origins and how the diverse phenomena associated with this condition have been viewed from ancient times until today.

Preface

The more people this book captures, the more it will have reached its goal. "Understanding Tourette Syndrome" is not "only" this new title in the Routledge *Understanding Atypical Development* book series, it is also an actual matter within health and social contexts, thus involving millions of subjects – clinicians working in Neurology, Psychiatry, Neuroscience and Psychology departments, and most of all patients and caregivers. Without also forgetting paediatricians, general practitioners and other specialists. School is another crucial "place" trying to understand and solve Tourette syndrome (TS) issues.

Manuals are often limited, being too simple or too complex, resulting in part of their readership being excluded from the benefit of learning something new. In these pages, the aim was to combine basic knowledge with scientific relevance to concrete indications for the management of our sufferers. The task has been hard and, as a result, what follows can sometimes appear cumbersome, or in other points obvious, depending on readers' expertise.

Homogeneity is another controversy when exploring Tourette syndrome. First, because of the complexity of phenomenology and treatment during the development of the child. Second, the involvement of so many professional figures seems to divide topics into many branches. Teamwork is the solution for restoring the unique approach to the syndrome, in both the research field and while "caring and curing" a patient.

The authors are thankful above all to Professor James Frederick Leckman, chief of Yale Child Study Center, where the Tic Disorder & Obsessive-Compulsive Center is based. Thanks to his day-by-day clinical, research, academic and missionary work, Tourette syndrome is now understood by those people who live close to sufferers and by those who, previously, had never heard about it. Having a Foreword by James Leckman gives emphasis to the following chapters as he supported the authors while expressing that TS extends far beyond "having tics".

The authors' decades-long experience at Milan Tourette Syndrome Centre, alongside children, teenagers and adult patients, enables them to observe the syndrome and its evolution. The positive development of tic symptoms with age is confirmed. Other specialists, namely neurophysiologists, functional neurosurgeons, and radiologists collaborate at the Centre to expand the research area as much as possible.

The authors thank Roberta Galentino for the pluriannual collaboration as clinical and research psychologist and for her commitment in dealing with TS families.

Among the Functional Neurosurgery team, authors are thankful to Alberto Riccardo Bona and his chief, Professor Domenico Servello. Readers need to know that invasive treatments are rare, and they are not applied to children, only to a few selected adults.

Thank you also to Matteo Briguglio, who realised what has been suggested in the volume "The Second Brain" (1999), i.e. studying the co-influence between the intestine and the brain (Gershon MD. 1999. *The Second Brain*. New York, NY, USA. Harper Collins Publishers Inc.).

Selenia Greco and Donatella Comasini collaborated with authors by giving psychological support in Southern Italy, and by handling the political-organisational functions respectively.

Authors appreciate the everyday work of the youngest of us, and promising psychologist, Thomas Spalletti in helping the drawing-up and design of the text.

Professor Alessandro Antonietti, Head of Psychology Department at the University of Milan, introduced authors to Routledge's series. Mauro Porta and Carlotta Zanaboni Dina are thankful to Professor Antonietti, Routledge and Taylor & Francis Group for making possible the creation of this book.

Authors are grateful to Professor Davide Dèttore, Head of the Master Course in Clinical and Health Psychology and Neuropsychology at the University of Florence and renowned expert of obsessive-compulsive spectrum, for contributing to the supervision of the clinical cases.

The author (CZD) would like to personally thank Antilla and Dario for their continual guidance. Their friendship has been fundamental in realising this project.

To whom is the volume dedicated? To our patients. Each day they are enriching us from a human and from a scientific prospective. Being in touch with a person suffering from Tourette syndrome is a stirring life lesson.

English Proofreader: Antilla M. Pellei Holden.
Graphic Designer: Cecilia Spalletti.

Abbreviations

ADHD	Attention-Deficit/Hyperactivity Disorder
CBCL 4–18	Child Behavior Checklist for ages 4–18
CBT	Cognitive Behavioural Therapy
CNS	central nervous system
CY-BOCS	Children's Yale-Brown Obsessive Compulsive Scale
DBS	Deep Brain Stimulation
DSM-5	Diagnostic and Statistical Manual of Mental Disorders-fifth edition
ERP	Exposure and Response Prevention
GABA	γ-aminobutyric acid
GT	Georges Albert Édouard Brutus Gilles de la Tourette
HRT	Habit Reversal Training
ICD-10	International Statistical Classification of Diseases and Related Health Problems – tenth revision
NOSI	Non-Obscene Socially Inappropriate behaviours
OCB	Obsessive-Compulsive Behaviour
OC component	OCB/OCD/OCS
OCD	Obsessive-Compulsive Disorder
OCS	Obsessive-Compulsive Symptoms
PANS	Paediatric Acute-onset Neuropsychiatric Syndrome
PANDAS	Paediatric Autoimmune Neuropsychiatric Disorders Associated with group A beta-haemolytic Streptococcal Infections
PNS	peripheral nervous system
QoL	Quality of Life
SIB	Self-Injurious Behaviour
SSRIs	Selective Serotonin Reuptake Inhibitors
TS	Tourette syndrome
Y-BOCS	Yale-Brown Obsessive Compulsive Scale
YGTSS	Yale Global Tic Severity Scale

Chapter 1

A short history of Tourette syndrome*

Summary

In 1825, Itard first described a Tourette syndrome (TS) case: la Marquise de Dampierre having coprolalia and other behavioural diseases. In the second half of the 19th century, Gilles de la Tourette – a disciple of Charcot at the Salpêtrière Hospital – studied nine patients, giving the name to the syndrome. Between the 19th and the 20th centuries, the organic versus psychological origin of TS was debated. Nowadays, from the USA to Europe, it is considered a neurodevelopmental disease characterised not only by tics, but also by behavioural symptoms. Living with the syndrome has specific sociocultural implications.

Introduction

This chapter illustrates cultural panorama at the times of the syndrome's birth. TS has a centuries-old history (Figure 1.1).

The syndrome's name originates from Georges Albert Édouard Brutus Gilles de la Tourette (born 1857 Saint-Gervais-les-Trois-Clochers; died 1904 Lausanne), a French neurologist who lived

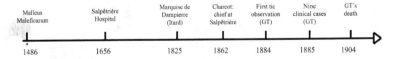

Figure 1.1 **Tourette's timeline.**
GT = Gilles de la Tourette.
Credit: Cecilia Spalletti.

---

* In collaboration with Thomas Spalletti

in a key period for development of medical sciences, especially neurology. He was born in Saint-Gervais into a family of doctors. In 1884, he started to follow the clinical practice of the Father of Neurology, Jean-Martin Charcot at the Salpêtrière Hospital. In 1885, Gilles de la Tourette (GT) published his studies on a bizarre disease in Charcot's "Archives de neurologie" (transl. "Archives of neurology"). He described nine cases affected by multiple tics, especially involving the face, superiority in the arts, and uncontrollable verbal bursts, including insults and profanities. The first case – the Dampierre Marquise – appeared 60 years earlier in the "Archives générales de médecine" (transl. "General archives of medicine", 1825) by the well-known doctor, Jean Marc Gaspard Itard. He made an accurate description of the case, and GT chose it as an emblem of the pathology that he called "la maladie de tics" (transl. "the tic disease"). Charcot then named the disease "Gilles de la Tourette syndrome", in honour of his pupil.

In 1886, GT graduated; in 1887, he became clinical head and his career grew. In 1893, GT was shot by a patient who was convinced to be in a state of hypnosis; the man tried to get out the state and fired three gunshots. The young neurologist suffered from brain damage, and his studies started to decline. After some years of medico-legal consultations, he became head doctor at Paris 1990's Expo. Then he contracted syphilis and he recovered in Lausanne, where he died at the age of 46, abandoned by his wife and whole family. GT's clinical notes on the syndrome are still valid today.

Early descriptions

GT was not the first doctor to be interested in the disease. He put together several clinical signs of this unique syndrome, thanks to other clinicians' case observations.

Previous descriptions of the disorder belong to different eras. The most ancient dates back to the age of inquisitors: the "Malleus Maleficarum" (transl. "The Witch Hammer", 1486), a text drawn up by two Dominican monks, Krämer and Sprenger. At that time, Pope Innocenzo VIII enacted a strict intervention against witchcraft, considering it a form of Satanism. In the aforementioned text, some cases are defined as demonic possessions, but many signs are now attributable to TS. One case is about the story of a Bohemian farmer, who went to Rome to ask his son – a priest – to free him from his demonic possession. Each time he stood in front of a church, the devil took possession of his tongue, and the man started to curse God and to swear. In those moments he couldn't control his words. Finally, a bishop took care of him through prayer, exorcism and by feeding him only bread and water for 50 days; then the man was graced by God and he could go back home.

Demonic manifestation was the best way to interpret this pathology, characterised by violent movements, shouts and lack of control. This case has a positive ending, whereas many others could have ended under torture.

Origin of the word "tic"

"Tic" has an onomatopoeic origin in different languages: *tic* in French and Italian, *tico* in Spanish, *tic/tik/tug* in English, *zucken/ziehen/zugen/tucken/ticket/tick* in German dialects.

The term was used for the first time in veterinary medicine to describe horses' pathologic breathing. From 1664, Solleysel, a well-known squire at Versailles, prevented buyers from purchasing horses with tics. The sound "tic" comes from the noise a horse makes when it hits the wood of the stable with its teeth. This happens when a horse is bothered by air in its stomach. Despite not being a contagious disease, horses learn it from each other (see echopraxia in Chapter 3).

La Marquise de Dampierre

La Marquise de Dampierre was a noblewoman, as described by Itard, and 60 years later by GT in his article. This was published a few months after the Marquise's death, i.e. when she was 85 years old. She was famous not only for being a Marquise, but also for her bizarre behaviour, which caused surprise and rumours.

At the age of 7, she had onset symptoms: severe mouth, face, neck and arm tics. Shouts, insults and obscenity bursts appeared some years later. Because of these problems, the noblewoman spent her life segregated in her palace until her death. Her speech would suddenly be interrupted with shouts, swearing and unexpected words, despite her high intelligence and good manners. When she was with other people, she used to inappropriately describe others,

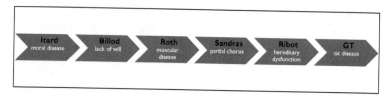

Figure 1.2 Interpretation of Marquise's symptoms.
GT = Gilles de la Tourette.
Credit: Cecilia Spalletti.

causing embarrassment to all the bystanders. The more she was scandalised by her own explicitness and by the repetition of these vulgarities, the more these words were "forced" onto her tongue, and she couldn't control herself.

Besides Itard and Gilles de la Tourette, many other clinicians tried to examine the Marquise's clinical conditions (Porta & Sironi, 2016; Figure 1.2). The point of view of each doctor follows:

1   **Itard** (1825) interpreted the Marquise's clinical case under the influence of the philosopher de Condillac, who believed that learning depends on sensorial stimulation. Based on this hypothesis, Itard assumed that a sufferer could overcome their disorder through a "moral treatment", a re-education training focused on force of will and emotions, offering senses stimulation. Health status depended on the balance of diet, weather conditions, job and lifestyle. Itard supposed that the Marquise was not able to exercise her will on behaviours as she was passively accepting her social role of wife and lady (e.g. her husband decided she wouldn't be cured). An appropriate intervention would have comprised of increasing her self-esteem. Many doctors at that time hypothesised that the frequent female diseases were the result of women's alienation forced upon them by their role in a patriarchal culture. This female arrest could be solved by improving women's life conditions through the development of a higher sensibility (in some cases, it would have been necessary for the patient to live away from her pathogenic home temporarily).

2   **Billod** (1847) identified the Marquise's poor will as the reason for expressing those thoughts, which would have normally been

suppressed. In contrast to Itard, Billod described the will as an entity, which can't be treated by a rehabilitation of the senses. Billod believed that a sane intellect can select ideas to express or not to express at all. In the Marquise's case, this ability would have been altered because her will was being absorbed by other influences.

3   Roth (1850) referred to the Marquise, rejecting both Itard's and Billod's interpretation. He supposed that her symptoms were caused by a physiologic cause: a muscular disease, namely chorea. He considered swearing and vocal bursts as "muscular tics of the word and the larynx".

4   Sandras (1851) defined the Marquise's symptoms as organic, i.e. being a partial chorea.

5   Ribot (1883) employed the Degeneration Theory to explain the Marquise's case. This theory was used to interpret many diseases (depression, intellectual disability, sterility, etc.) as consequences of bad moral and social behaviour, along with hereditary features. Alcohol abuse, an unbalanced diet and immoral actions would have disruptive effects on the nervous system, whose cerebral alterations would be transmitted down through generations.

6   Gilles de la Tourette (1885) illustrated the Marquise as being Charcot's patient. Despite this, his master never visited the woman. Charcot knew about his pupil's interest towards tics and the bizarre cases reported from Malesia, Siberia and Maine (e.g. startle, swearing, imitation and other behaviours). GT created a connection between these behaviours, and patients with tics hospitalised at the Salpêtrière Hospital, and he first identified the syndrome. The Father of Neurology pushed GT to deal with this unclear pathology, taking advantage of the medical fame of Charcot himself.

It is remarkable that so many doctors, referring only to Itard's reports, provided such different interpretations! Finally, the Marquise case became the cornerstone of a wide range of pathologies.

Charcot at the Salpêtrière Hospital

Jean-Martin Charcot was the biggest figure in the medical world in the 19th century. Born in 1825 in Paris and the son of a cart manufacturer, Charcot was initially doubtful about his own career.

He first conducted both medical and artistic studies, then he started his clinical activity in his town as assistant doctor at the Salpêtrière Hospital. After a long training period, in 1862 he became head; in the following decades, he transformed the decadent Parisian hospital into a prestigious and internationally renowned neurological centre (Porta & Sironi, 2016).

The history of the hospital

The origin of the Pitiè-Salpêtrière dates back to 1544. It was a Christian poorhouse for the care of those who were infirm in body or spirit.

After few decades, a state reform converted the charity centre into a care centre for acute treatable patients (and no longer for people with chronic conditions, as in the medieval epoch). Many hospitals were built in Europe, marking the changeover from charity to healthcare. Even so, it was still necessary to guarantee a place for poor people and assistance for chronic patients. For this reason, in 1656 King Louis XIV established the General Hospital of Paris with many departments located in the town. The Salpêtrière Hospital started to take care of the poor, sick people, cripples, orphans, elderly people and prostitutes.

Over the years, the number of sufferers admitted to the Salpêtrière Hospital grew: from 628 people in 1657 to around 8,000 in 1788.

At the end of 18th century, Pinel and Esquirol – the Fathers of Psychiatry – introduced a healthcare reform, giving dignity back to mental illness patients who were currently alienated in dedicated facilities. The Salpêtrière Hospital was converted into a mental health hospital.

Some years later, the hospital become a clinical research unit thanks to the great number of patients, and the first electrophysiological and neuropathological studies were conducted there. Its photographic centre could also record the hospital's historical evolution of nervous and mental illness.

Tourette: neurological or psychiatric disease?

Following Descartes' dualism between body and mind (Descartes, 1637), neurological diseases (organic alteration of the nervous system) should be unrelated to psychiatric diseases (mental disorders). Charcot was inspired by this separation, when he figured out that diseases are mostly caused by organic or mental features.

At the Salpêtrière Hospital, he observed either neurological and psychiatric manifestations. Charcot started his studies on multiple sclerosis, Parkinson's disease, epilepsy and other diseases. He was principally renowned for his studies on hysteria and hypnosis. In 1870, he became head of the Epileptic Women Unit, and he realised that not all the patients with epileptic symptoms were suffering from epilepsy. Some of them presented no neurological alterations, and he started to consider them as being affected by hysteria. In 1881, he depicted hysterical functioning, and the use of hypnosis in enhancing its symptoms.

Charcot became more and more renowned, and he was exposing his research to students and colleagues at the "Leçons du Mardi" (transl. "Tuesday Lessons"). Sigmund Freud took also part in his lessons about Psychoanalytic Theory.

In 1882, he became chair of the first Nervous System Diseases' university department.

Between 1885 and 1890, he studied tics, illustrating the results in lectures. Tics were attributed to a fully psychic origin. They were considered as recurrent, involuntary and complex movements, without purpose (i.e. they were compared to a caricature of normal behaviours). Tics' purposelessness was the reason to consider them as having a psychic origin, despite the organic nature of their manifestations.

After centuries of debating – largely in Europe and in USA – the diatribe is now resolved: TS is considered a neurological disorder with behavioural implications (cf. 2011's European Guidelines). Still, the ancient dualism – together with a social stigma towards psychiatric diseases – influences today's society.

Gilles de la Tourette, MD

GT's observations of tics date back to 1884. He mentioned three clinical conditions suggesting a unique disease, and being strictly related, with tics (Gilles de la Tourette, 1884): the American "Jumping", the Malaysian "Latah" and the Siberian "Myriachit". Details on these phenomena and two European cases are as follows:

- The American neurologist Beard (1882) reported some cases he observed in Maine. They were characterised by nervousness and abnormal motor responses to external stimuli. Sound or visual solicitations elicited jumping, and the repeated execution of any task that was firmly asked. The *Jumping* syndrome was observed in American families, native French and transferred in Maine. Beard described the case of a man who was cutting his tobacco with a knife, when someone suddenly shouted at him, "throw it!": the man immediately and repeatedly threw the knife, sticking it in a door.

- Two years later, O'Brien (1884), a non-medical observer, depicted similar phenomena occurring in Malaysia and Bangladesh. In Asia it was called *Latah*, and it could manifest in two ways. The first one was – as for Jumping – the automatic and involuntary execution of a suddenly shouted order, with a startled reaction and jumping. The second one was the same, but without motor alterations. O'Brien mentioned the case of a ship's cook, holding his baby on the ship's bridge, cradling him. A sailor started to joke by cradling a log wrapped in a cloth, and suddenly threw it towards the bridge. The cook was watching, and immediately replicated the action; he unintentionally threw his baby on the ground and killed him.
- Hammond (1884) illustrated a comparable behaviour between the Siberians, naming it *Myriachit*. The author described a Russian army captain, while crossing a river, making fun of a boatman because he couldn't resist imitating anything he watched or heard (e.g. grunting, clapping, hopping).
- In Germany the disease was called *Schafftzunkenheit*: in this case the person was woken up by someone who was suddenly commanding a task. The subject would execute the task, even if asked to kill someone.
- A French 15-year-old boy was affected by head and upper body tics and startles, repeated the cursing "s**t" and the words that he heard.

These cases show complex behavioural alterations often accompanied by tics, which are the two main components of TS.

In 1885, Gilles de la Tourette described and published for the first time nine clinical cases, starting with the Dampierre Marquise case (cf. Table 1.1). He observed six of these cases; the remaining three cases have been described by other doctors.

As Charcot was renowned for having distinguished epilepsy from hysteria, GT was notorious for having defined "La Maladie des Tics Convulsifs" (transl. "Convulsive Tic Disorder") in the

Table 1.1 GT's nine cases and symptoms (definitions are in Chapter 3). Patients are presented following the original order.

Sex	Age	Tics' body area (motor tics; sound tics)
F (the Dampierre Marquise)	26	mouth, face, neck and arms; coprolalia
M	20	head, arms and legs; coprolalia and other sound tics
M	15	grimaces, head, neck, arms and shoulders, walking and other motor tics; coprolalia
M	24	face, limbs, jumping (when it is raining), walking and other motor tics; echolalia, palilalia
M	14	eye, SIB (biting lips), grimaces, limbs, jumping; sound tics
M	11	eye, grimaces and other motor tics; sound tics
M	21	eye, walking and other motor tics; sound tics
F	15	shoulders and other motor tics; animal imitation, coprolalia and other sound tics
M	24	SIB (biting tongue), limbs and other motor tics; coprolalia, palilalia

F= female; M= male.
SIB= Self-Injurious Behaviour (cf. Chapter 3).

homonymous article (Gilles de la Tourette, 1899). He considered it a complex syndrome, with no moral but psychic origin. GT's findings received such a great support from Charcot that the Father of Neurology renamed the syndrome in honour of his pupil.

Latest findings

The 20th century conceived many approaches and theories for studying human behaviour. Interest in the mind and its connection to the body and physical health was growing when psychoanalysis made its way into the medical world. Sigmund Freud was the Father of this new discipline; his heirs integrated his theory, sometimes altering it. For many years, psychoanalytic interpretations of tics dominated on the scene (Figure 1.3), and they were seen as the expression of a suppressed libido. Tics represent an outburst as the result of suppression, and they were even hypothesised to be the surrogate of masturbation.

Later, psychoanalytic theories about tics have been disproved by medical findings. In 1968, the spouses Arthur and Elaine Shapiro published a key article (Shapiro & Shapiro, 1968), which changed the perspective on tics. They demonstrated the organic origin of tics and the inefficacy of psychoanalytic therapy: they successfully treated a patient with haloperidol, a neuroleptic drug (Figure 1.3). In the article, they reported the clinical case, emphasising the neurological origin of TS, and the efficacy of organic therapies against the psychoanalytic approach. The Shapiros' finding transformed TS' vision and encouraged new evidence-based studies.

In recent decades (Van Woert et al, 1976; Carroll & Robertson, 2000), a genetic component has been revealed as another cause of

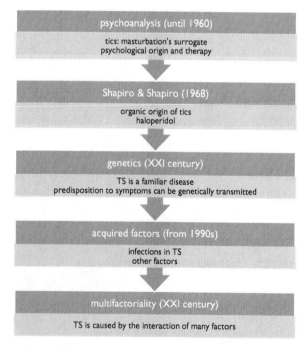

Figure 1.3 From the psychoanalytic to the multifactorial TS view.
Credit: Cecilia Spalletti.

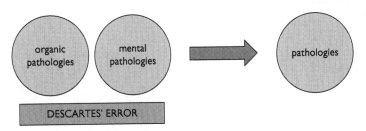

Figure 1.4 From the Descartes' error to the holistic view of pathologies.
Credit: Cecilia Spalletti.

TS, considering the high probability of transmitting symptoms to offspring (Figure 1.3; cf. Chapter 2). The familiar predisposition had already been assumed by GT, but only the modern genetic techniques allowed ad hoc research.

Recently (Allen et al, 1995), the organic view of TS has been confirmed by its frequent correlation with infections and other acquired factors (Figure 1.3; cf. Chapter 2). These studies make clear that the syndrome has multifactorial and interacting causes (Figure 1.3; cf. Chapter 2).

Scientific progress has led to a refusal of the dualism of body/mind, introduced by Descartes centuries ago: the two entities interact in human beings. The reciprocity between brain and mind brings together organic and mental pathologies towards a holistic view of pathologies (Figure 1.4). TS represents both components: symptoms have an organic origin and manifestation, but they are influenced by psychological factors (Robertson, 2000; Roessner et al, 2011).

Conclusions

In ancient times, TS attracted great curiosity because of the singularity of its symptoms and has generated beliefs related to the spirit. In the last centuries, scientific progress has increased medical knowledge about the syndrome. Today, ongoing studies are increasing the understanding of its complex causes, symptoms and treatments. In the next chapters, the main scientific findings about TS will be exposed to clarify the nature of the syndrome and how sufferers, families and other people involved can approach this fascinating phenomenon.

References

Allen AJ, Leonard HL, & Swedo SE. 1995. Case study: A new infection-triggered, autoimmune subtype of pediatric OCD and Tourette's syndrome. Vol 34(3). *Journal of the American Academy of Child & Adolescent Psychiatry*, 307–311.

Beard GM. 1882. *Study of Trance, Muscle-Reading and Allied Nervous Phenomena in Europe and America, With a Letter on the Moral Character of Trance Subjects, and a Defence of Dr. Charcot.* New York, NY, USA: LA University of California.

Billod E. 1847. Des maladies de la volonté, ou études des lesions de cette faculté dans l'aliénation mentale. In: *Annales médico-psychologiques.* Geneva, CH, EU: L. Martinet.

Carroll A & Robertson M. 2000. *Tourette Syndrome: A Practical Guide for Teachers, Parents and Carers.* New York, NY, USA: David Fulton Publishers, 5.

Descartes R. 1637. *Discours de la méthode.* Leiden, NL, EU: Ian Maire.

de la Tourette G. GAÉB. 1884. Jumping, Latah, Myriachit. Vol 8. *Archives de neurologie.* Paris, FR, EU: Bureaux du progrés medical, 68–74.

de la Tourette G. GAÉB. 1885. Étude sur une affection nerveuse caractèrisée par de l'incoordination motrice accompagnée d'écholalie et de copro-lalie (jumping, latah, myriachit). Vol 9. In: Charcot JM, ed. *Archives de neurologie.* Paris, FR, EU: Bureaux du progrés médical, 19–42 and 158–200.

de la Tourette, G. GAÉB. 1899. La maladie des tics convulsifs. Vol 19. *La semaine médicale*, 153–156.

Hammond WA. 1884. Myriachit: Newly described disease of nervous system and its analogues. Vol 39. *New York Medical Journal*, 191–192.

Itard JMG. 1825. Mémoire sur quelques fonctions involontaires des appareils de la locomotion, de la préhension et de la voix. In: *Archives Générales de Médecine.* Paris, FR, EU: Béchet, 385–407.

Krämer HI & Sprenger J. 1486. *Malleus maleficarum.* Strasbourg, FR, EU.

O'Brien HA. 1884. Latah. Vol 12. *Journal of the Straits Branch of the Royal Asiatic Society*, 283–284.

Porta M & Sironi A. 2016. *Il cervello irriverente. La sindrome di Tourette, la malattia dei mille tic.* Bari, IT, EU: Ed. Laterza, 9–21.

Ribot T. 1883. *Les maladies de la volonté.* Paris, FR, EU: Felix Alcan.

Robertson MM. 2000. Tourette syndrome, associated conditions and the complexities of treatment. Vol 123(3). *Brain*, 425–462. Review.

Roessner V, Rothenberger A, Rickards H, & Hoekstra PJ. 2011. European clinical guidelines for Tourette syndrome and other tic disorders. Vol 20(4). *European Child & Adolescent Psychiatry*, 153–154.

Roth D. 1850. *Histoire de la musculation irreésistible ou de la chorée anormale.* Paris, FR, EU: JB Baillère.

Sandras CMS. 1851. *Traité pratique des maladie nerveuses*. Vol 2. Paris, FR, EU: Germer-Baillière, 518–519, 522–523 and 528.

Shapiro AK & Shapiro E. 1968. Treatment of Gilles de la Tourette's Syndrome with haloperidol. Vol 114(508). *British Journal of Psychiatry*, 345–350.

Solleysel J. 1664. *Le parfait maréchal*. Paris, FR, EU.

Van Woert MH, Jutkowitz R, Rosenbaum D, & Bowers MB Jr. 1976. Gilles de la Tourette's syndrome: Biochemical approaches. Vol 55. *Research Publications – Association for Research in Nervous and Mental Disease*, 459–465.

Chapter 2

A medical overview of Tourette syndrome*

Summary

Tourette syndrome (TS) can be considered a sensory-sensitive brain disorder with a motor circuit dysfunction, producing tics and behavioural diseases. The pathological mechanism consists of a dysfunction of the cortico-striato-thalamo-cortical circuit. Many neurotransmitters (dopamine, serotonin, γ-aminobutyric acid and others) also play a role in the pathological mechanism, and this could explain the symptoms' variation.

The main causes of the syndrome include: a) genetics and b) acquired factors (perinatal problems and infections). With regards to infections, similar dysfunctions are involved in TS, Obsessive-Compulsive Disorder, and Paediatric Autoimmune Neuropsychiatric Disorders Associated with group A beta-haemolytic Streptococcal Infections.

More genetic, neuroimaging, neurophysiology and neuropathology studies are needed to clarify the TS mechanism and to optimise the diagnostic-therapeutic process.

Introduction

Medical bases of TS are presented to the readers to help them classify TS as an organic disease. TS originates from genetics and other medical factors, such as infections. On the other hand, many disciplines are involved in the syndrome, thus requiring teamwork. TS team is usually composed by medical doctors (neurologist, psychiatrist, and occasionally, neurosurgeon), psychologists and psychotherapists, family doctors and other specialists e.g. dietician (see Box 2.1).

* In collaboration with Matteo Briguglio

> ## Box 2.1   TS patients need teamwork to be managed
>
> ### TS team of clinicians
>
> - medical doctor (neurologist/psychiatrist/neurosurgeon)
> - psychologist/psychotherapist
> - family doctor
> - other specialists

Despite the necessity of such a team of specialists, an official certification for TS experts still doesn't exist.

Brain anatomy, movement and behaviour

In this section, the most relevant brain aspects (Blundo, 2004) to understand tics and TS behavioural symptoms are introduced.

The *brain* is the complex structure (approximate weight: 1.3 kg) where movements, sensations, memories, thoughts, words and emotions arise. It is the central organ of the *nervous system* (composed by the central and peripheral nervous system). The nervous system receives, selects and processes stimuli coming from inside and outside the body (Figure 2.1).

The *central nervous system* (CNS; Figure 2.2) is divided into the brain and the spinal cord. The CNS is made of agglomerates of grey matter (neurons) and white matter (tissue connecting different areas of grey matter).

The *peripheral nervous system (PNS)* is made of nerves and groups of nerves, called ganglia, located outside the brain and the spinal cord. Its main function is exchanging information between the CNS and the rest of the body. It is dived into: *somatic nervous system* – responsible for voluntary responses – and *autonomic nervous system* –responsible for involuntary responses.

Cranial nerves are the nerves emerging from the brain and belonging to the PNS. They relay information primarily from and to regions of the head and the neck. They regulate motor and sensory functions, such as:

- hearing and balance
- vision

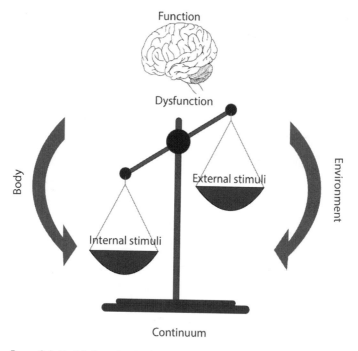

Figure 2.1 Brain's function in the continuum between internal and external stimuli (modified from Blundo, 2004).

Credit: Cecilia Spalletti.

- smell
- taste
- face sensitivity
- face movement

Spinal nerves belong to the PNS too, but they emerge from the spinal cord. They relay information from and to the remaining body areas (i.e. torso and limbs), having a motor-sensory function.

Neurons (approximately 86 billion) hold information inside the brain, they are connected by the release of substances called neurotransmitters (e.g. dopamine, serotonin, noradrenaline, GABA and acetylcholine). Motor neurons, for instance, are connected to muscles by acetylcholine. Tics are determined by an alteration of dopamine and other neurotransmitters (cf. the next paragraph).

Specific neurotransmitters activate also the *autonomic nervous system*, which is the regulator of visceral functions through stimuli coming from internal organs e.g. heart, liver and intestine. This system controls also other functions such as piloerection, salivation and the so-called "fight-or-flight" response i.e. the physiological defence in front of a danger (see also Chapter 4).

The spinal cord is connected to the brain through the *brain stem*, a fundamental structure which is middle-positioned, laterally and under the cerebellum. This is the pathway for all the sensory and motor connections. Evolutionally, the brain stem is the nervous system's more archaic portion.

The *cerebellum*, as well, is one of the more ancient structures of the nervous system. It is located behind the brain stem, under the brain mass, and it is the main responsible for learning and coordination of complex movements (e.g. walking). Its work is similar to a boat's stabiliser, without it the hull would be at the waves' mercy.

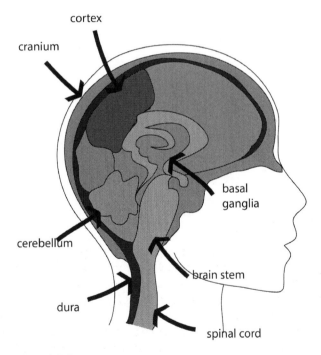

Figure 2.2 Brain components.
Credit: Cecilia Spalletti.

The brain is made up of two areas: *diencephalon* and *telencephalon*. The diencephalon is composed of different structures, including the thalamus and hypothalamus.

The *thalamus* is considered as a "transit and sorting station" of a) sensory, b) motor and c) behavioural information. The *hypothalamus*, positioned in the centre under the thalamus, is composed of grey matter nuclei with a homeostatic function, i.e. the maintenance of adaptive body conditions to both external and internal states. The hypothalamus controls the autonomic nervous system by regulating: sense of appetite, body temperature, sleep-wake cycle and other essential functions.

The thalamus and hypothalamus are connected to the *limbic system*. This system is made of the CNS' interacting structures. The latter are not responsible for "what to do" but for the related emotions (e.g. fear or aggressiveness) and memories, influencing the "how/when" of doing something. The limbic system regulates impulses and behaviours linked to these self-conservative mechanisms: smell, reproduction and care for offspring, nutrition, motivation and self-consciousness. The limbic system also connects the autonomic nervous system and the neuroendocrine system, i.e. the system responsible for hormone secretion in the brain.

For 1) movement regulation, 2) movement-related emotions and 3) motor learning, basal ganglia have a key role (Figure 2.3). Basal ganglia are altered in tics (cf. the next paragraph). They are the following grey matter substances, placed under the cortex, in the left and right part of the brain:

- striatum, composed by:
  - caudate nucleus
  - putamen
  - nucleus accumbens
  - olfactory tubercule

- globus pallidus
- ventral pallidum
- substantia nigra
- subthalamic nucleus

Basal ganglia belong to the "extrapyramidal system" (in contrast to the cortical voluntary "pyramidal system", so-called because of

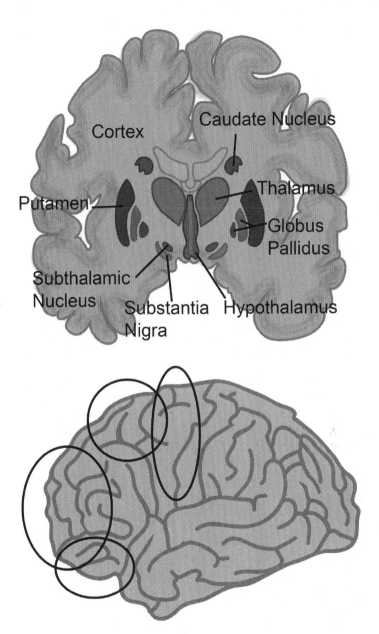

Figure 2.3 Basal ganglia – on the top – regulates movements. Tics are determined by an altered basal ganglia functioning – involved circuits on the bottom.

the pyramidal-shaped nervous cells), interchanging with the cortex and the thalamus.

The *cortex* regulates the "superior activities" e.g. attention, awareness and thought. In the motor and premotor cortical areas, fine voluntary movements (e.g. precise hand movements) are planned (as a robot-like action), and then executed. Basal ganglia have two main functions:

1   smoothing voluntary movements
2   controlling involuntary movements

In this regard, Jankovic (1997) classifies movements in four types (Table 2.1): voluntary, semivoluntary (or unvoluntary), involuntary and automatic. The first ones are intentional (planned, self-initiated, internally generated) or responsive movements (induced by external stimuli). Semivoluntary movements are induced by both inner sensory stimuli (cf. tics' premonitory urge in the next paragraph) or feelings (especially obsessions in TS). Automatic movements are unintentional (e.g. walking and speaking). Tics don't belong to a unique type, they range from being semivoluntary to automatic, thus including involuntary movements (see Table 2.1). These latter can be suppressible as usually tics or tremors are, or insuppressible as in case of reflexes.

Both motor and sound tics are anticipated by the so-called *premonitory urge* or premonitory sensation (Cohen & Leckman, 1992): a physical/psychological urgency, which signals the tic arrival. It is

Table 2.1 Modified from Jankovic's classification of movements (1997).

Voluntary	–
intentional	
responsive to external stimuli	
Semivoluntary (Unvoluntary)	TIC
induced by inner sensory stimuli	
induced by feelings/obsessions	
Involuntary	TIC
insuppressible (e.g. reflex)	
suppressible (e.g. tremor)	
Automatic	TIC
learned without conscious effort (e.g. walking)	

present in 90% of cases (Leckman et al, 1993), and it is perceived after 10 years of age (Leckman et al, 1998). Premonitory urge, even if not always present or perceived, is a crucial element for the TS diagnosis. Patients describe the physical urge, being located in the same body area of tics or in others, as:

- discomfort/incompleteness
- a need to move
- a sense of pressure
- a sense of cold or warm
- a tingle
- a tickle
- a shiver

The psychological urge is an obsession, which can precede tics or compulsions. For example, an obsession with fingernails being perfect can lead to a nail biting tic.

Inside the pyramidal cortex, it is possible to draw the "homunculus motorius" and the "homunculus sensorius" (see Figure 2.4). Hands, limbs and face are largely represented in the former, thus having a finer motility than other body areas. In the latter, hands, feet and mouth are largely represented, thus indicating that these areas have the higher sensibility. The two homunculi could explain the reason of a major tic's activation in these areas. TS is indeed considered a "sensory-sensitive" dysfunction, and not only a motor dysfunction (cf. also sensorial and sensitive features in Chapters 3 and 7).

In short, the nervous system can't be considered as a sum of distinct areas: it is a complex system constantly processing data, in which each area works together with the others.

Tourette syndrome is the result of an alteration of both organic and mental functioning. Brain structures analyse body signals, recognising them sometimes as sensations, and sometimes as emotions, and therefore producing behaviours. It's impossible to separate the study of brain functions from the study of the body. People that do, reiterate Descartes' error (see Chapter 1). Understanding the mind implies a holistic view of human nature.

Considering these bases of anatomy and functioning of the nervous system, TS can be classified as an "organic" disease having psychopathological implications.

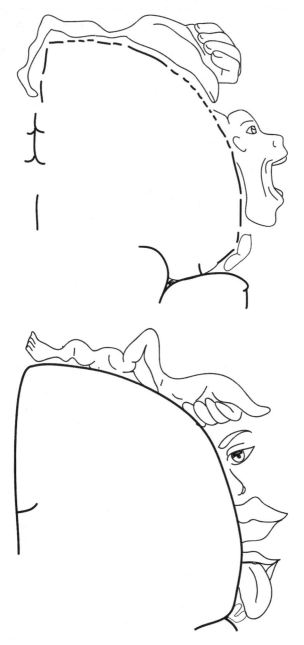

Figure 2.4 Homunculus motorius (2.4, top) and homunculus sensorius (2.4, bottom).

Credit: Cecilia Spalletti.

TS brain features: pathophysiology

Pathophysiology studies the mechanisms underlying diseases, including anatomical alterations and dysfunctions – in this case, of the brain. In order to provide insights into the pathophysiology of TS, different studies have been conducted (Thenganatt & Jankovic, 2016); further results are yet to be found, especially those regarding anatomical alterations.

Alert!

Tics result from dysfunction in the cortico-striato-thalamo-cortical circuit.

Dopamine and other neurotransmitters are involved in TS, as well.

Structural and functional neuroimaging studies (see "functional magnetic resonance" in the Glossary) define TS as a network disorder with dysfunction not only of the extrapyramidal system, but also of other cortical and subcortical regions, namely of the sensorimotor cortico-striato-thalamo-cortical circuit (Leckman et al, 2010; Worbe et al, 2015a). Some authors (Worbe et al, 2015b; Robertson, 2015) suggest that cortical abnormalities are related to tics' premonitory urges. Leckman et al (2010) have also described preliminary results on abnormalities in the limbic and other circuits. Current research is focused on:

- *depth and thickness of grey matter* in some cortical areas and in the caudate nucleus is reduced and associated with tic severity (Muellner et al, 2015; Robertson, 2015). It is unclear if this is a neuropathological cause or consequence. Cortical and subcortical regions are linked by the phenomenon of connectivity.
- *connectivity* (i.e. patterns of links in the brain) of cortical and subcortical regions is reduced and associated with tic severity (Church et al, 2009; Cheng et al, 2013; Zapparoli et al, 2017). These findings are in line with the framework of TS as a disorder of brain immaturity during the neurodevelopmental process.

- *plasticity* (i.e. ability of the brain to change and adapt to experience) of the cortex (Brandt et al, 2014), basal ganglia and brain stem (Suppa et al, 2014) is abnormal. This mechanism could alter the TS motor control processing.
- *neurotransmitters* (cf. previous paragraph). Dopamine is the main one implicated in TS, but serotonin, noradrenaline, γ-aminobutyric acid (i.e. GABA), glutamate and acetylcholine are also determinant (Udvardi et al, 2013). Other unidentified neurotransmitters could be relevant too (Porta & Sironi, 2016).
- *microglia* (i.e. cells located in the brain and in the spinal cord with the role of immune protectors). Recently (Vaccarino et al, 2013), the effect of a dysfunction in microglia is stressed in TS pathophysiology. It also directly relates to the reduced patterns of neuronal connectivity listed earlier.

Pathophysiology, together with etiopathology (see the next paragraph), contributes to the study of diagnosis (see Chapter 3) and treatment (see Chapter 4).

TS causes: etiopathology

Etiopathology studies the causes of pathologies. Regarding Tourette syndrome, two principal causes must be analysed: genetics and acquired factors (Figure 2.5).

Genetics

Genetic factors are significant in determining TS (Deng et al, 2012). TS is a family disorder:

- Each TS sufferer has a 55% possibility to transmit to his child a genetic predisposition to TS features, namely tics, OCB, ADHD (Carroll & Robertson, 2000).
- The heritability depends by the degree of genetic relatedness: First-degree relatives are more likely to transmit a genetic predisposition than second-degree relatives, who in their turn more likely transmit it than third-degree relatives (Mataix-Cols et al, 2015).
- In 25% of cases, both parents of the sufferer are affected (Hanna et al, 1999).

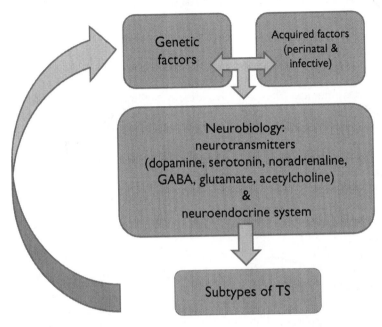

Figure 2.5 Causes of TS, and their influence on subtypes.
Credit: Cecilia Spalletti.

Between the different genetic studies in TS (Fernandez et al, 2018), many authors have been focused on the mutation of the gene SLITRK1 (Abelson et al, 2005; Karagiannidis et al, 2012) and of the gene histidine decarboxylase (Ercan-Sencicek et al, 2010; Pittenger, 2017).

In TS patients, genetic factors interact with neurobiological factors, i.e. neurotransmitters and the neuroendocrine system, thus differentiating the symptomatology expressed in each subtype (Figure 2.5; for subtypes cf. Chapter 3). Regarding the neuroendocrine system, stress steroid hormones and the oxytocin hormone could be implicated in TS (Martino et al, 2013).

No blood tests are available for TS predictive diagnosis. Parents often ask for a consultation with specialists before pregnancy. Clinicians can only offer a consultation based on statistical data.

More genetic studies, also considering the different TS subtypes (Chapter 3), are needed.

Acquired factors

With less evidence than genetics, acquired factors are the other etiopathological element. Genetics and acquired factors can be coexistent. Genetics strictly determine the presence/absence of the syndrome, acquired factors increase vulnerability ("meiopragia" in medicine) to develop TS. The main acquired factors are:

1   perinatal factors
2   infections

Perinatal factors in TS (Robertson, 2000; Santangelo et al, 1994) include:

- severe nausea/vomiting during pregnancy, and medications to prevent it.
- birth complications, for example the umbilical cord around the baby's neck, jaundice (i.e. pathology whose main symptoms are yellowish skin pigmentation and eyes), prematurity (i.e. baby being born at 36 weeks of gestation or earlier), Caesarean section, forceps delivery and a prolonged labour.
- foetal excessive exposure to either caffeine, tobacco, or alcohol increases Obsessive-Compulsive Disorder vulnerability (cf. OCD in Chapter 3).

Infections is the second acquired factor. The immune system is the one dealing with infections; when it is activated it protects the body.

"Paediatric Autoimmune Neuropsychiatric Disorders Associated with group A beta-haemolytic Streptococcal Infections" (PANDAS) is a spectrum of TS-like acute symptoms, belonging to "Paediatric Acute-onset Neuropsychiatric Syndrome" diseases' group (PANS). It results from the activation of the brain antibodies after Group A Streptococcus infections (Swedo et al, 1998; Martino et al, 2011). Neuroimmunologic studies on TS, OCD and PANDAS have established that a similar immune dysregulation contributes to the pathophysiology of the three disorders; a better understanding of the mechanism is still needed.

Alert!

Infections play the same role in TS, OCD and PANDAS!

One possible immunologic common element are microglia (Frick & Pittenger, 2016). Microglial dysregulation in TS, OCD and PANDAS has the same roots –including inflammatory process in the striatum (Morer et al, 2010; Kumar et al, 2015) – and it can be both cause and consequence of the three diseases.

PANDAS/TS studies are linked to the microbiota studies. Gut microbiota is the population of microorganisms that colonize the gut, including bacteria, fungi and viruses. It contributes in metabolism, intestinal barrier function and prevention of pathogenic colonisations. Alterations in the gut microbiota are possibly participating in PANDAS/TS spectrum because of the interconnections between gut, microbiota and brain (Petra et al, 2015). For all these links between PANDAS and TS, the authors speculate PANDAS being a TS subtype (see also Chapter 3).

TS etiopathological research influences subtypes (Figure 2.5). Based on the studies of Robertson (2000), Dell'Osso et al (2017) proposes OCTD as the TS subtype given by the overlap of TS and OCD symptoms (see details in Chapter 3). The union of these pathologies would increase the epidemiological data of TS patients, i.e. the number of sufferers.

Other studies are analysing the role of:

1   mirror neurons in TS. These neurons "mirror" the actions and behaviours of others. Rationale (Rizzolatti & Fogassi, 2014; Bandura, 1971) refers to learning tics/TS behaviours from other people. Ecophenomena (i.e. the repetition of someone else's words or movements; it must be out of context) is an example of typical TS mirror-like symptom.

2   seasonality in TS. Many disorders, such as cluster headache (i.e. a type of headache), follow a periodical trend during the year. According to the clinical experience of the authors, there could be a link between TS symptoms' wax-and-waning and seasonality. The authors speculate that sensory

responsible of these variations in TS, for example,
during summer may represent one trigger of tics'
ion.

ns

TS pathophysiology and etiopathology have implications onto the diagnostic-therapeutic process.

Today, no TS examinations are available to predict or confirm the diagnosis, nor to clarify the prognosis. The following lab examinations guide the treatment (cf. Chapter 4):

- *pharyngeal swab and blood examinations*, including streptococcal infection index (i.e. Antistreptolysin O titer). Results can confirm the infective etiology in TS patients. In some cases, caregivers are also required to have their own streptococcal infection examinations, as they can be infection holders.
- *electrocardiogram* to guarantee a safe drug intaking.
- *gut microbiota test*. This has recently started to be used in TS Centres.
- *nuclear magnetic resonance* to exclude other pathologies.
- *other more specific examinations* are sometimes used.

The international Tourette syndrome's associations promote meetings and global studies to identify new findings in the understanding of the pathophysiology and etiopathology of TS.

Alert!

Patients and caregivers can help the research by taking part in study trials.

References

Abelson JF, Kwan KY, O'Roak BJ, Baek DY, Stillman AA, Morgan TM, ..., & State MW. 2005. Sequence variants in SLITRK1 are associated with Tourette's syndrome. Vol 310. *Science*, 317–320.

Bandura A. 1971. *Social Learning Theory*. New York, NY, USA: General Learning Press, 1016.

Blundo C. 2004. *Neuropsichiatria: I disturbi del comportamento tra neurologia e psichiatria.* Milano, IT, EU: Masson, 3–20, 63–132, 239–278.

Brandt VC, Niessen E, Ganos C, Kahl U, Bäumer T, & Münchau A. 2014. Altered synaptic plasticity in Tourette's syndrome and its relationship to motor skill learning. Vol 9(5). *PLoS One,* e98417.

Carroll A & Robertson M. 2000. *Tourette Syndrome: A Practical Guide for Teachers, Parents and Carers.* New York, NY, USA: David Fulton Publishers, 5.

Cheng B, Braass H, Ganos C, Treszl A, Biermann-Ruben K, Hummel FC, . . . , & Thomalla G. 2013. Altered intrahemispheric structural connectivity in Gilles de la Tourette syndrome. Vol 4. *Neuroimage,* 174–181.

Church JA, Fair DA, Dosenbach NU, Cohen AL, Miezin FM, Petersen SE, & Schlaggar BL. 2009. Control networks in paediatric Tourette syndrome show immature and anomalous patterns of functional connectivity. Vol 132(1). *Brain,* 225–238.

Cohen AJ & Leckman JF. 1992. Sensory phenomena associated with Gilles de la Tourette's syndrome. Vol 53. *Journal of Clinical Psychiatry,* 319–323.

Deng H, Gao K, & Jankovic J. 2012. The genetics of Tourette syndrome. Vol 8(4). *Nature Reviews Neurology,* 203–213.

Dell'Osso B, Marazziti D, Albert U, Pallanti S, Gambini O, Tundo A, . . . , & Porta M. 2017. Parsing the phenotype of obsessive-compulsive tic disorder (OCTD): A multidisciplinary consensus. Vol 21(2). *International Journal of Psychiatry in Clinical Practice,* 156–159.

Ercan-Sencicek AG, Stillman AA, Ghosh AK, Bilguvar K, O'Roak BJ, Mason CE, . . . , & State MW. 2010. L-histidine decarboxylase and Tourette's syndrome. Vol 362. *New England Journal of Medicine,* 1901–1908.

Fernandez TV, State MW, & Pittenger C. 2018. Tourette disorder and other tic disorders. Vol 47. *Handbook of Clinical Neurology,* 343–354.

Frick L & Pittenger C. 2016. Microglial Dysregulation in OCD, Tourette Syndrome, and PANDAS. *Journal of Immunology Research,* doi: 10.1155/2016/8606057.

Hanna PA, Janjua FN, Contant CF, & Jankovic J. 1999. Bilineal transmission in Tourette syndrome. Vol 53(4). *Neurology,* 813–818.

Jankovic J. 1997. Tourette syndrome: Phenomenology and classification of tics. Vol 15(2). *Neurologic Clinics,* 267–275. Review.

Karagiannidis I, Rizzo R, Tarnok Z, Wolanczyk T, Hebebrand J, Nöthen MM, . . . , & Paschou P. 2012. Replication of association between a SLITRK1 haplotype and Tourette Syndrome in a large sample of families. Vol 17(7). *Molecular Psychiatry,* 665–668.

Kumar A, Williams MT, & Chugani HT. 2015. Evaluation of basal ganglia and thalamic inflammation in children with pediatric autoimmune neuropsychiatric disorders associated with streptococcal infection and tourette syndrome: A positron emission tomographic (PET) study using 11C-[R]-PK11195. Vol 30(6). *Journal of Child Neurology*, 749–756.

Leckman JF, Walker DE, & Cohen DJ. 1993. Premonitory urges in Tourette's syndrome. Vol 150. *American Journal of Psychiatry*, 98–102.

Leckman JF, Zhang H, Vitale A, Lahnin F, Lynch K, Bondi C, . . . , & Peterson BS. 1998. Course of tic severity in Tourette syndrome: The first two decades. Vol 102. *Pediatrics*, 14–19.

Leckman JF, Bloch MH, Smith ME, Larabi D, & Hampson M. 2010. Neurobiological substrates of Tourette's disorder. Vol 20(4). *Journal of Child and Adolescent Psychopharmacology*, 237–247.

Martino D, Chiarotti F, Buttiglione M, Cardona F, Creti R, Nardocci N, . . . , & Italian Tourette Syndrome Study Group. 2011. The relationship between group A streptococcal infections and Tourette syndrome: A study on a large service-based cohort. Vol 53(10). *Developmental Medicine & Child Neurology*, 951–917.

Martino D, Macerollo A, & Leckman JF. 2013. Neuroendocrine aspects of Tourette syndrome. Vol 112. *International Review of Neurobiology*, 239–279.

Mataix-Cols D, Isomura K, Pérez-Vigil A, Chang Z, Rück C, Larsson KJ, . . . , & Lichtenstein P. 2015. Familial risks of Tourette syndrome and chronic tic disorders: A population-based cohort study. Vol 72(8). *JAMA Psychiatry*, 787–793.

Morer A, Chae W, Henegariu O, Bothwell AL, Leckman JF, & Kawikova I. 2010. Elevated expression of MCP-1, IL-2 and PTPR-N in basal ganglia of Tourette syndrome cases. Vol 24(7). *Brain, Behaviour and Immunity*, 1069–1073.

Muellner J, Delmaire C, Valabrégue R, Schüpbach M, Mangin JF, Vidailhet M, . . . , & Worbe Y. 2015. Altered structure of cortical sulci in gilles de la Tourette syndrome: Further support for abnormal brain development. Vol 30(5). *Movement Disorders*, 655–661.

Petra AI, Panagiotidou S, Hatziagelaki E, Stewart JM, Conti P, & Theoharides TC. 2015. Gut-microbiota-brain axis and its effect on neuropsychiatric disorders with suspected immune dysregulation. Vol 37(5). *Clinical Therapeutics*, 984–995.

Pittenger C. 2017. Histidine decarboxylase knockout mice as a model of the pathophysiology of Tourette syndrome and related conditions. In: Y Hattori, R Seifert, eds. 2017. *Handbook of experimental pharmacology: Histamine and histamine receptors in health and disease*. Berlin, GE, EU: Springer-Verlag, 189–215.

Porta M & Sironi A. 2016. *Il cervello irriverente: La sindrome di Tourette, la malattia dei mille tic*. Bari, IT, EU: Ed. Laterza, 132–141.

Rizzolatti G & Fogassi L. 2014. The mirror mechanism: Recent findings and perspectives. Vol 369(1644). *Philosophical Transactions of the Royal Society London B Biological Science*. doi: 10.1098/rstb.2013.0420.

Robertson MM. 2000. Tourette syndrome, associated conditions and the complexities of treatment. Vol 123(3). *Brain*, 425–462. Review.

Robertson MM. 2015. A personal 35 year perspective on Gilles de la Tourette syndrome: Assessment, investigations, and management. Vol 2(1). *Lancet Psychiatry*, 88–104.

Santangelo SL, Pauls DL, Goldstein JM, Faraone SV, Tsuang MT, & Leckman JF. 1994. Tourette's syndrome: What are the influences of gender and comorbid obsessive-compulsive disorder? Vol 33(6). *Journal of the American Academy of Child & Adolescent Psychiatry*, 795–804.

Suppa A, Marsili L, Di Stasio F, Berardelli I, Roselli V, Pasquini M, . . . , & Berardelli A. 2014. Cortical and brainstem plasticity in Tourette syndrome and obsessive-compulsive disorder. Vol 29(12). *Movement Disorders*, 1523–1531.

Swedo SE, Leonard HL, Garvey M, Mittleman B, Allen AJ, Perlmutter S, . . . , & Dubbert BK. 1998. Pediatric autoimmune neuropsychiatric disorders associated with streptococcal infections: Clinical description of the first 50 cases. Vol 155(2). *American Journal of Psychiatry*, 264–271.

Thenganatt MA & Jankovic J. 2016. Recent Advances in Understanding and Managing Tourette Syndrome. Vol 5. *F1000Research*. doi: 10.12688/f1000research.7424.1.

Udvardi PT, Nespoli E, Rizzo F, Hengerer B, & Ludolph AG. 2013. Nondopaminergic neurotransmission in the pathophysiology of Tourette syndrome. Vol 112. *International Review of Neurobiology*, 95–130.

Vaccarino FM, Kataoka-Sasaki Y, & Lennington JB. 2013. Cellular and molecular pathology in Tourette syndrome. In: Martino D & Leckman JF, eds. *Tourette Syndrome*. Oxford, UK, EU: Oxford University Press, 205–220.

Worbe Y, Marrakchi-Kacem L, Lecomte S, Valabregue R, Poupon F, Guevara P, . . . , & Poupon C. 2015a. Altered structural connectivity of cortico-striato-pallido-thalamic networks in Gilles de la Tourette syndrome. Vol 138(2). *Brain*, 472–482.

Worbe Y, Lehericy S, & Hartmann A. 2015b. Neuroimaging of tic genesis: Present status and future perspectives. Vol 30(9). *Movement Disorders*, 1179–1183.

Zapparoli L, Tettamanti M, Porta M, Zerbi A, Servello D, Banfi G, & Paulesu E. 2017. A tug of war: Antagonistic effective connectivity patterns over the motor cortex and the severity of motor symptoms in Gilles de la Tourette syndrome. Vol 46(6). *European Journal of Neuroscience*, 2203–2213.

Chapter 3

Diagnosing Tourette syndrome

Summary

Tourette syndrome's diagnosis is based on the presence of tics – motor and at least one sound tic – before 18–21 years old and for at least a year. Behavioural diseases accompany tics; the main ones are Attention-Deficit/Hyperactivity Disorder and obsessive-compulsive (OC) component. Both tics and behavioural diseases vary during the life of the sufferer.

The method used for diagnosing the syndrome consists of a neuropsychiatric visit to a doctor together with various clinical scales to complete. The main scales are the Yale Global Tic Severity Scale, the Yale-Brown Obsessive Compulsive Scale and other specific scales to assess Attention-Deficit/Hyperactivity Disorder, depression, anxiety symptoms and Social Impairment.

Tourette syndrome (TS) may manifest itself as five or more subtypes, thus inviting stakeholders to gradually talk in terms of "Tourette syndromes" rather than "Tourette syndrome".

Few prognostic reports are outlined here, as scientific data are still limited at this time of writing.

Introduction

Diagnosis is the first medical phase every patient needs to cope with. This chapter aims to provide the essential elements to TS patients and caregivers in order to prepare them for their first visits to a doctor. They will be interviewed and observed by the doctor. When the diagnosis is given, they will be elucidated about TS' broad spectrum of symptoms, both neurological and behavioural. Considerations about what to expect for the future clinical condition of the child are outlined at the end of the chapter.

A good TS team usually uses the information that follows in this chapter to ensure a correct understanding of that particular TS patient, the specific subtype and specific level of Social Impairment.

Diagnostic criteria

TS is defined by the worldwide-used manual "Diagnostic and Statistical Manual of Mental Disorders-fifth edition" (DSM-5 cf. APA, 2013; Table 3.1) as a neurodevelopmental disorder characterised by more than a motor tic and at least a sound tic. Age of onset should be before 18 (21 according to The Tourette Syndrome Classification Study Group, 1993). N.B. often, adult patients had tics in childhood, but do not recall them. When tics onset in adulthood, they are caused by other medical conditions and they are called "secondary adult-onset tics".

DSM-5 also defines Other Tic Disorders, i.e. Persistent Tic Motor or Vocal Disorders (Table 3.2) if just motor or sound tics

Table 3.1 Adapted from DSM-5 diagnostic criteria for Tourette syndrome.

DSM-5: Tourette syndrome

A. more than a motor tic and at least a sound tic has been present during the pathology, not necessarily concurrently.
B. tics may wax and wane in frequency, but they have lasted for more than one year since the onset.
C. onset is before age 18.
D. the disorder is not caused by the effects of a substance (e.g. cocaine) or other medical conditions (e.g. Huntington's disease).

Table 3.2 Adapted from DSM-5 diagnostic criteria for Persistent Motor or Vocal Tic Disorder.

DSM-5: Persistent Tic Disorder

one or more motor tics or one or more sound tics, but not both motor and sound ones.
N.B. The doctor must specify in the diagnosis whether the disorder exists with motor or sound tics.
the tic/s may wax-and-wane but has/have lasted for more than one year since first onset.
the tic/tics started before 18 years old.
symptoms are not caused by any medicines/drugs or by other medical conditions (e.g. post-viral encephalitis).
absence of Tourette syndrome diagnosis.

Table 3.3 Adapted from DSM-5 diagnostic criteria for Provisional Tic Disorder.

DSM-5: Provisional Tic Disorder
one or more motor tics and/or one or more sound tics.
the tic/s has/have lasted for less than one year.
the tic/tics started before 18 years old.
symptoms are not caused by any medicines/drugs or by other medical conditions (e.g. post-viral encephalitis).
absence of Tourette syndrome diagnosis and Persistent Tic Disorder diagnosis.

are present, and Provisional Tic Disorder (Table 3.3) if tics are present for less than a year.

The other well-known manual, "International Statistical Classification of Diseases and Related Health Problems-tenth revision" (ICD-10 cf. World Health Organization, 2003), specifies that tics may be present many times a day, almost daily; whereas DMS-5 does not refer to tic frequency (see Table 3.1).

ICD-10 only – differently from DSM-5 – includes an impairment criterion. ICD-10 underlines that no treatment is needed if the patient has no impairment with his everyday life. The author (CZD) agrees, if the patient can judge his own impairment (see adequate IQ and global mental integrity). In case of Self-Injurious Behaviour or suicidal thoughts, the doctor will decide on a treatment to preserve the patient's safety.

Neither manual includes biological markers. This makes it harder to get to a correct diagnosis! The worldwide scientific committee is trying to identify these markers to facilitate the diagnostic process.

The prevalence of Tourette syndrome is higher than the prevalence of other Tic Disorders. In the majority of TS Centres, DSM-5 is more used than ICD-10.

Spectrum of the syndrome and prevalences

TS prevalence is up to 1% of the population (Robertson, 2015); this datum reaches 18–20% in children and adolescents (Bloch & Leckman, 2009). TS is more common in males than in females (3–4 times more common in males) and less common in people of sub-Saharan black African, African-American, and American Hispanic ethnic origins (Robertson, 2015).

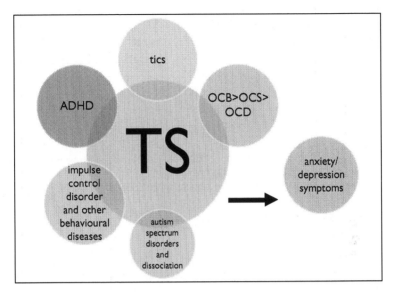

Figure 3.1 The broad spectrum of TS symptoms.
Credit: Cecilia Spalletti.

Several people – including many doctors – are not aware of these data, and consequently the syndrome is underdiagnosed. If including patients with obsessions and compulsions>tics and patients with PANDAS (their features are explained in the following paragraphs) the percentage increases considerably.

Readers should know that TS is characterised not only by tics, but by a wide spectrum of behavioural symptoms associated with tics, as well (Robertson, 2000; Figure 3.1).

Tics are repetitive, nonrhythmic and purposeless movements, they may be motor tics (e.g. blinking) or sound tics (e.g. coughing).

Tics can be classified into:

- *Clonic tics* i.e. quick, snap movements (e.g. blinking).
- *Dystonic tics* i.e. slower than clonic tics, miming dysfunctional postures (e.g. teeth grinding).
- *Tonic tics* i.e. slower than dystonic tics, progressive muscular contraction (e.g. arm stretching).

Tics may vary in relation with:

- *Typology* i.e. type of movement or of sound. Every movement or sound can become a tic.
- *Complexity* i.e. from a simple tic involving just one or two body parts at the same exact moment (e.g. eye blinking) to a pattern of tics involving many body parts at the same exact moment (e.g. eye blinking plus shoulder scrolling plus sniffing).
- *Frequency* i.e. from once a day tic to recurrent tics (=every few seconds).
- *Intensity* i.e. the same typology of tic (e.g. eye blinking) could be from slight to very marked.
- *Interference* i.e. the quantity of tic interference with other activities (e.g. homework).
- *Social Impairment* i.e. from an absence of discomfort to severe forms of isolation.

In childhood, tics are located in the face or head area, in adolescence/adulthood they gradually move to the body periphery i.e. legs and arms (Figure 3.2).

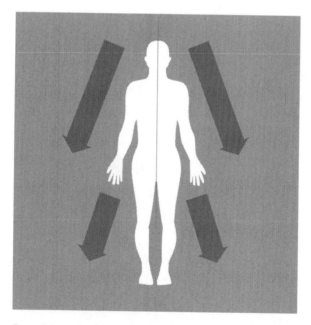

Figure 3.2 Evolution of tics from childhood towards adulthood.
Credit: Cecilia Spalletti.

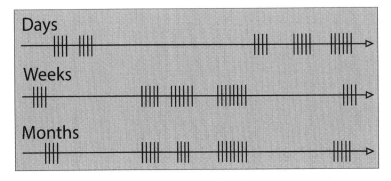

Figure 3.3 Bouts of tics during days/weeks/months, adapted from Leckman and Cohen (1999).
Credit: Cecilia Spalletti.

Tics appear in "bouts" (Leckman & Cohen, 1999), i.e. the patient has daily, monthly, yearly tic attacks as tics are not stable, but they wax-and-wane (Figure 3.3). Bouts occur especially in childhood, whereas in adulthood tics become chronic and more stable.

The DSM-5 (APA, 2013) definition of tics as "motor movement" needs further explanation. Every movement is, indeed, motor; furthermore, it is antiquated to separate motor and sound tics as every sound tic needs a movement in order to be realised. Moreover, authors prefer to call them "sound" tics and not "vocal" tics because voice is not always involved (e.g. in the case of sniffing or coughing).

As better explained in Chapter 2, we recall that tics are anticipated by the "premonitory urge", a physical/psychological sensation that signals the arrival of a tic. Premonitory urge is fundamental for the differential diagnosis as it is a marker of TS, even if diagnostic manuals still do not consider it as being so.

The following are definitions of the most complex tics that a TS person may have:

- *Coprolalia*: repetition of obscene word/s or sentences, they must be out of context.
- *Copropraxia*: repetition of obscene movements, they must be out of context.
- *Echolalia*: repetition of someone else's word/s, they must be out of context.

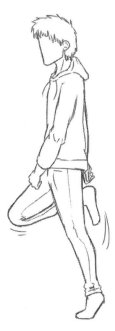

Figure 3.4 Examples of handwriting (top) and walking tics (bottom).
Credit: Cecilia Spalletti.

- *Echopraxia*: repetition of someone else's movements, they must be out of context.
- *Palilalia*: repetition of one's own utterance/s, they must be out of context.
- *Handwriting tics*: paligraphia i.e. writing again and again the same letter/word/sentence (for instance "today today today is a sunny day d d d d"), outlining each letter multiple times (Figure 3.4), and pulling the pen back while writing (Zanaboni Dina et al, 2016).
- *Walking tics* (see Figure 3.4): leg tics while walking (for instance to lift a leg or to drag feet while walking or to take a step forward and two back).
- *Non-Obscene Socially Inappropriate behaviours (NOSI)*: inappropriate behaviours or tics (e.g. shouting out "bomb" in an airport). They are related to the impulsivity of the TS sufferer and they could have serious social consequences.
- *Stuttering*: speech with involuntary disruptions such as repetitions of sounds/syllables/words, or prolongation of sounds, or interruptions of speech.
- *Change in the tone of voice*: it manifests randomly, not only in relation to emotional changes.

Psychogenic (or functional) tics are tics with a psychological cause. For example, a child could deliberately (or not) make a nose wrinkle because he understands that every time he makes it his parents give him attention that he wouldn't otherwise receive. The consciousness of the tic action doesn't make a difference in considering the tic a functional one: the child can be conscious or unconscious of the tic and its consequence, and in both cases this tic is considered functional.

Malignant tics are painful tics. An example could be the pain caused by a frequent neck roll tic.

Self-Injurious Behaviour (SIB) is self-harm without intention of death; its prevalence in TS is 33% (Robertson et al, 1989). Every part of the body may be damaged by tics, in some cases, severely (paraplegia for example). As for physical aggression, SIB requires therapy even if the person is opposed to it.

Comorbidities

Table 3.4 lists TS comorbidities, i.e. highly concomitant pathologies with TS. It has to be stressed that tics and comorbidities have the same origin because they share the genetic background (cf. Chapter 2).

Table 3.4 Percentages of comorbidities in TS.

Comorbidity	% of comorbidity
Attention-Deficit/Hyperactivity Disorder	59–60% (Rothenberger & Roessner, 2013)
Obsessive-Compulsive Behaviour	11–80% (Robertson, 1989)
Obsessive-Compulsive Symptoms	
Obsessive Compulsive Disorder	
Impulse Control Disorder (and rage)	23–40% (Wright et al, 2012)
Autism Spectrum Disorders and dissociation	6.5–10% (Baron-Cohen et al, 1999; Porta & Sironi, 2017)

In order of prevalence, of course *Attention-Deficit/Hyperactivity Disorder (ADHD)* is the most common – around 59 to 60% of comorbidity (Table 3.4). This disorder can include: attention deficit and/or hyperactivity-impulsivity (APA, 2013).

Attention deficit is not, really, a lack of attention, but a hyperactivation of the attention process itself. It is, indeed, a control deficit. The absence of control means not being able to select the important stimuli while inhibiting the unimportant ones.

The attention deficit component in TS often increases because of tics/obsessions/compulsions (e.g. a child loses his attention while reading because of an eye blinking tic), or by the fact that the sufferer focuses all the attention on controlling tics/obsessions/compulsions (Morand-Beaulieu et al, 2017).

As a result, the TS person may (Morand-Beaulieu et al, 2017):

- have deficits in maintaining the attention on one or multiple targets (attention deficit component).
- show purposeless movements and behaviours aiming to relieve an inner tension (hyperactive component).
- act without considering consequences (impulsive component).

Usually, ADHD is first noticed by school teachers during lessons (see Figure 3.5): the student can't stay seated for long and he continuously moves in the classroom or outside (hyperactive component); he has a short attention span during lessons or homework (attention deficit component); and he struggles to wait (impulsive component).

Other examples of attention deficit component:

- switching from one activity to another and leaving tasks unfinished.
- difficulty in organising or processing information.
- missing details, forgetting or losing things.
- becoming easily confused or bored of a task within a short space of time.
- daydreaming.

Other examples of hyperactive-impulsive component:

- squirming and fidgeting while seated.
- making inappropriate comments or manifesting emotions without reservation.
- interrupting conversations or others' activities.

N.B. An ADHD diagnosis requires symptoms to be present before 12 years old and in at least two contexts, usually at school and at home (APA, 2013).

In TS, ADHD represents the first phase of the disorder, around 5 years of age.

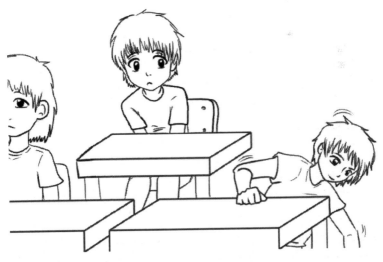

Figure 3.5 School is one of the principal settings in which to start collecting data to diagnose ADHD.

Credit: Cecilia Spalletti.

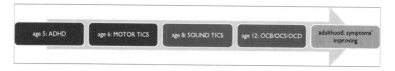

age 5: ADHD   age 6: MOTOR TICS   age 8: SOUND TICS   age 12: OCB/OCS/OCD   adulthood: symptoms' improving

Figure 3.6 Evolution of symptoms in TS from childhood towards adulthood.
Credit: Cecilia Spalletti.

After the first years of ADHD, at around 6–7 years old, the first motor tics appear and they are followed by sound tics at around age 8 (Figure 3.6). Ultimately, obsessions and compulsions arrive in late childhood/adolescence i.e. around 12 years old and can become the most permanent and impairing pathology in TS (Figure 3.6). The worst period for TS patients is considered to be when they are 10 to 12 years old (Jankovic & Kurlan, 2011). Adults improve in 50–75% of cases (Bloch, 2013). In the remaining cases, they maintain obsessions and compulsions>tics>ADHD.

Obsessive-Compulsive Behaviour (OCB)/ Obsessive-Compulsive Symptoms (OCS)/ Obsessive-Compulsive Disorder (OCD) (i.e. OC component) are present in 11 to 80% of TS patients (Table 3.4); because of this high prevalence, it has been recently coined the TS subtype "Obsessive-Compulsive Tic Disorder" (see paragraph, "Subtypes").

OC component is made of behaviours (i.e. actions are pathological, whereas thoughts are intact), symptoms (traits and not a global disorder) or disorders (global disorder with pathological thoughts and actions) characterised by purposeless thoughts and actions.

Regarding thoughts, "obsessions" is the term for the symptoms. Obsessions are intrusive, undesired repetitive ideas, or images of a specific object, which can be a living being or inanimate. They can be accompanied by feelings of fear or annoyance or disgust. "Compulsions" are, instead, repetitive undesired actions (or thoughts), used by the patient to block obsessions. An example of obsession is the disgust for germs, and the relative compulsion can be repetitive hand washing.

Considering typologies, almost every idea and behaviour may become an obsession or compulsion. The most common OC typologies in TS are related to the 5 senses (e.g. touching objects while watching them or finding specific sounds irritating) or they

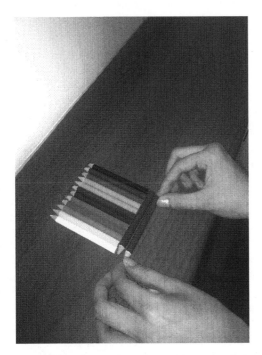

Figure 3.7 Compulsion of symmetry.

are related to the following themes: order, symmetry (Figure 3.7), aggressiveness, repetition, controls, body image and hygiene.

The following are definitions of the complex OC features that a patient may have:

- *Trichotillomania or hair pulling disorder*: the urge to pull out one's hair. The person usually has a preferred area of hair pulling e.g. head or genitals or beard. It can be associated with trichophagia (eating the pulled hair). Trichophagia can lead to trichobezoar (a hairball in the gastrointestinal system), which requires surgery.
- *Avoidances*: the avoidance of the actions/people/objects/places linked with one's own obsessions or compulsions. For example, the sufferer will avoid cinemas if he is obsessed by cinema seat germs.

- *Mental rituals*: the compulsion for which the patient repeats one or more word/sentence in his head.
- *Caregivers' involvement in rituals*: the involvement of a caregiver in the person's rituals. The aim is to have accomplices/helpers. For example, Giovanni asks his mother to repetitively clean his laundry because he is obsessed by cleanliness. The pathology is often expanded to many family members.
- *Perfectionism*: the obsession of making or thinking or feeling everything in a flawless way. It is accompanied by critical self-evaluation (particularly when a performance has not reached the high standard the person was seeking), and by concerns regarding others' opinion.
- *Obsessive doubt*: it is the pathological doubt. It leads to rumination, control and repetitions of actions, and therefore, time wasting. A classic example for a child could be the obsession with forgetting a specific book at home, this child could compulsively check in the bag to see if he has the book with him at school. Eventually, because of his obsession. the child could continuously put the book in or take it out of the bag. Paradoxically, as a self-fulfilling prophecy, finally he could even forget the book.
- *Obsessive slowness*: the behaviour of someone who carries out everyday activities in an extremely slow manner. An example is a person taking 30 minutes to wash their face. It may manifest also in the inability to quickly inhibit an action to move to a new one i.e. cognitive-behavioural rigidity in front of change. An example could be the unexpected change of school schedule (Maths instead of English class): a TS child would continue and be focused on the habitual class (English).
- *Magic thoughts*: the belief that something positive or negative will happen in relation with the sufferer's obsession and/or compulsion. Example of magic thought: "If I touch the desk three times I will get a great mark in Maths!"
- *Evening up*: the repetition of an action both to the left and to the right side because of an inner urge of the sufferer. For example, Charles sniffs both his left and right hand as compulsion, if he doesn't, he feels nervous.
- *Just right/Just so*: the repetition of an action in a subjective right manner, usually connected with a visuo-tactile sensation e.g. "I walk without stepping on the cracks between paving slabs because I feel fulfilled in this way".

The most common OC features in TS are: caregivers' involvement in rituals, perfectionism, obsessive doubt, evening up and the so-called just right.

> ## Alert!
>
> Caregivers may be involved in rituals:
>
> Do not adhere to the patient's rituals by explaining the reason.

Impulse control disorder is present in 23–40% of TS patients (Table 3.4). It may include, in order of frequency, from more frequent to less:

- intermittent explosive disorder (i.e. excessive outbursts of anger and violence; the involuntary nature of the aggression is clear when, after the episode, the patient feels guilty and apologises).
- compulsive buying (or shopping, which may be linked with Internet addiction).
- pathological gambling (more often in adult patients because of the law's restriction for its use in children).
- Internet addiction (i.e. excessive web surfing).
- kleptomania (i.e. stealing as the main pathological action).
- pyromania (i.e. setting things on fire as the main pathological action).
- sexual compulsion (i.e. pathological sexual attitude).

Impulse control disorder in children highly correlates with ADHD.

Impulsivity (Hollander & Rosen, 2000) may be considered a common element of all TS symptoms.

Autism spectrum disorder is a comorbid diagnosis in TS patients in 6.5% of cases (Table 3.4). It is a severe neurodevelopmental disorder, characterised by social communication and interaction deficits, and other cognitive-behavioural diseases.

Coexistent psychopathologies

Table 3.5 is a list of TS coexistent psychopathologies. Differently from TS comorbidities (=highly concomitant disorders), coexistent

Table 3.5 Percentages of coexistent psychopathologies in TS.

Coexistent psychopathologies	% of coexistence
Anxiety	45% (Erenberg et al, 1987)
Depression	13–76% (Robertson, 2006)
Sleep disorders	25% (Freeman et al, 2000)
Neurocognitive deficits	≈19% (Morand-Beaulieu et al, 2017)
Oppositional defiant disorder	14.5% (Robertson et al, 2015)
Personality disorder	51.5% (Trillini & Müller-Vahl, 2015)

psychopathologies may be concomitant disorders or consequences of having tics. Furthermore, in contrast to tics and comorbidities, tics and coexistent psychopathologies don't share the same genetic background.

Anxiety and depression are considered as the principal coexisting psychopathologies (Table 3.5). Anxiety is more common than depression symptoms (45% versus 13–76%, Table 3.5). Anxiety can manifest itself through general anxiety/preoccupation, phobias (e.g. school phobia) and panic attacks, whereas depression symptoms are usually expressed by rage attacks/low self-esteem in TS children and irritability/sadness/apathy/low self-esteem in TS adults.

Sleep disorders is another frequent (25%, Table 3.5) coexisting psychopathology for TS. Bedtime is one of the worst moments of the day for the patient as tics increase because of tiredness. During the day, the TS sufferer tries to control – consciously or not – tics, and at bedtime no energy is left. At night, different sleep problems may occur such as:

- night terrors (terror or dread while sleeping)
- insomnia
- sleep talking or walking
- nightmares
- bedwetting or bruxism or other tics

Neurocognitive deficits are quite common: ≈19% (Table 3.5).

In Tourette patients (especially with ADHD and/or OC component) the following elements may be present:

- association between high tic severity and memory deficits.
- slightly impaired fine and gross motor performance.

- lacking inhibitory system.
- poor academic achievement in maths.
- learning disorders such as dyslexia and dyscalculia.

Oppositional Defiant Disorder is quite common in TS (14.5% in Table 3.5; Figure 3.8), as well. The disorder's pattern includes rage/irritable mood, controversial behaviour, or revenge. A typical attitude of the oppositional defiant disorder sufferer is to start any sentence with "no".

It is prevalent when TS is comorbid with ADHD and when there is a family history of verbal and physical aggressiveness.

Personality disorder traits (= traits may be not pathological) are present in 51.5% of TS patients (Table 3.5). Personality Cluster C Disorder (i.e. obsessive-compulsive, avoidant, dependent) traits seem to be the most typical comorbid personality disorders in TS (Trillini & Müller-Vahl, 2015). Further studies underline that 15% of TS patients have a diagnosis of schizotypal personality disorder (Cavanna et al, 2007).

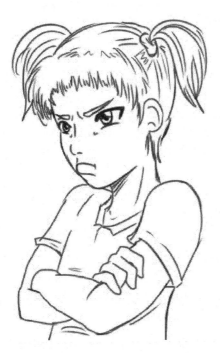

Figure 3.8 Sonia in a typical oppositional defiant disorder attitude.

N.B. As this book is principally dedicated to children, it must be specified that generally personality disorders can be diagnosed only after 18 years old (APA, 2013).

TS subtypes

According to Mary Robertson (2015), five Tourette syndrome subtypes may be recognised (Grados et al, 2008). They differ in the presence/absence of tics, OCB, OCD and ADHD. This classification comes from a study of 952 patients of the TS Association International Consortium on Genetics. The study underlines also that only the TS+OCD+ADHD subtype is highly heritable. Specific elements of this subtype (symmetry/exactness, aggressive urges, fear-of-harm, and hoarding) are being studied by Cath et al (in Hirschtritt et al, 2018).

This distinction of subtypes helps the reader to understand that TS is not a one-way disorder. Parents of TS children are usually worried about TS diagnosis because of the possibility to develop SIB, coprolalia and a high Social Impairment, but fortunately the spectrum is broad and mild cases may even require no treatment!

Of course, the TS+OCD+ADHD subtype could be the worst condition, but it always depends on the severity level of symptoms.

Obsessive-Compulsive Tic Disorder (OCTD) (Dell'Osso et al, 2017) is a modern classification of a TS subtype, which includes the OC component as principal feature together with tics. Robertson (2015), in the above-mentioned classification, outlines four out of five subtypes including OC component.

Precisely, OCTD subtype has been conceived by a group of TS and OCD experts (Dell'Osso et al, 2017) when they noticed that the two pathologies overlap each other. OCD patients have often been affected by tics, especially at a young age. The same goes for TS patients, often affected by OC component from adolescence onwards. Furthermore, repetitive behaviours are sometimes difficult to classify as either tics or compulsions, since they have features of both. From a biological perspective, the two disorders share the same genetics, neuroanatomy, neurochemistry and the post-infectious autoimmune component (cf. Chapter 2).

In 2017, the expert group held a consensus conference to describe OCTD main characteristics:

- prevalence of <1% of general population, early onset, male gender.
- five senses-related symptoms; obsessions of symmetry, exactness, aggressiveness, hoarding and sounds.
- high comorbidity with ADHD and impulsive behaviours.
- higher impairment compared to that of TS without the OC component.
- need of a medical treatment (see Chapter 4), together with ad hoc psychotherapy in a multi-professional team.

After this first publication, the expert group conducted different clinical studies on OCTD theme (e.g. Scalone et al, 2017).

Alert!

Considering the huge number of subtypes, it is preferable to talk about "Tourette syndromes" rather than "Tourette syndrome".

Paediatric Autoimmune Neuropsychiatric Disorders Associated with group A beta-haemolytic Streptococcal Infections (PANDAS; Swedo et al, 1998)

PANDAS is a childhood acute-onset spectrum of the following TS-like symptoms: tics including handwriting tics, OCD, bed-wetting, night terrors, learning disorders and separation-related anxiety. These symptoms may arise after streptococcal infections (cf. Chapter 2), and they occur in the form of severe attacks.

Authors speculate PANDAS being a TS subtype because it has similar symptomatology and neuroimmunologic implications to TS.

The first "proper" visit in Tourette syndrome

The first visit with a specialist is, in itself, a great success for patients. Still, they have to be encouraged by mass media (tv, radio, web) to consider scheduling a visit with a TS specialist. Some family doctors do not identify in these patients a possible neurodevelopmental problem, or they tend to minimise it. Consequently, sufferers are sent to the wrong specialist (e.g. a dermatologist if the child repetitively scratches his skin, or an oculist if the child continuously blinks), or they are told to wait as "tics go away with growth". This malpractice causes a delay between the syndrome's onset and the beginning of the diagnostic-therapeutic pathway (more than 5 years as a medium delay cf. Mol Debes et al, 2008; Scalone et al, 2017), with clear psychosocial implications for the patient.

Alert!

Ask for an early diagnosis.

Usually, during a first visit a doctor listens, queries and checks the patient before making a decision. Whereas, on the other side of the desk, a patient is expecting (often with worry) the doctor's examination. Conversely, the TS patient has manifestations, depending on many factors that are partially controllable. For instance, considering mild obsessions, the anamnesis can only be based on the description of the patient.

A good doctor knows that time is never enough to exhaustively assess a Tourette patient, especially with regard to behavioural diseases. So, what should you expect? First of all, a long interview is held by the TS team with the patient and the caregivers. Primarily, the interview concerns genetic predisposition (whether the mother and father, and other relatives, have ever being affected by tics or dysfunctional behaviours). And, it also regards the possible exposure to ß-haemolytic streptococcus group A (were there frequent sore throats, or tonsil or adenoid removals of the patient or of the caregivers?) as another factor causing TS. When necessary, the doctor prescribes a pharyngeal swab and a blood dose of the Antistreptolysin O titer (Müller et al, 2000; Martino et al, 2011; Martino et al, 2015). No other biological examinations are necessary for a TS diagnosis! Unless there are tics, the neurological examination in TS patients is usually normal. This is seen as good news for the patient who will not have to undertake many examinations, but not for clinicians who have no biological markers on which to build up the diagnosis (cf. paragraph, "Diagnostic criteria").

Moreover, the patients are asked to remember their age and mode at tic onset, as well as the awareness of premonitory sensations of tics (Woods et al, 2005), and of behaviours such as irritability and aggressiveness, attention deficits, hyperactivity and OC component (Goodman et al, 1989). Last but not least, the doctor asks the patient about their degree of Social Impairment given by symptoms.

Other questions are going to be asked – maybe about school or about the girlfriend i.e. "awkward" questions – as they will be good stress tests while the doctor carefully observes the patient.

During the visit, the patient should be seated without crossing their arms or legs, and not wearing bulky jackets or bags, as it would be easier for them to hold back tics. Furthermore, in order to distract the patient (and therefore to encourage tic appearance), the doctor will interview the caregivers first. Actually, a lot of information is learned from the most subtle sign of restlessness, even if in front of a doctor tics are less frequent and intense than usual.

During the first and control visits, validated scales (see paragraph, "Clinical scales") together with a psychological interview, may be administered in relation to the particular spectrum of that TS patient (cf. paragraph, "TS subtypes").

However, "significant" tic manifestations can only be observed with severe TS patients, when the sufferer's suppression of attacks is extremely complicated. In the majority of the cases, vice versa, the doctor can only use his experience and cunning to "provoke" tics. Many people with TS can hold back tics in an excellent way, and therefore having received a "referred Tourette" diagnosis (i.e. symptoms are not visible during the visit, but referred by the patient/caregiver). In addition, parents can sometimes be extremely apprehensive and exaggerate in reporting small movements or some insignificant "noises"!

So, be prepared to not see the sufferer comfortably seated and dressed on the medical bed; the patient will have to answer many questions and to tolerate the investigative eye of the doctor and the psychologist.

Clinical scales

During the first and follow-up visits, TS-specific scales are administered by experts. Caregivers must be present as well to help the doctor to define the diagnosis. Indeed, the patient themself (especially in case of young children) can have a low insight about his symptoms.

Table 3.6 provides a list of principal TS scales.

Table 3.6 Main used scales in TS.

Symptoms	Scale name	Scale acronym	Authors, year
TS features	Diagnostic Confidence Index	DCI	Robertson et al, 1999
Tics	Yale Global Tic Severity Scale	YGTSS	Leckman et al, 1989
	Tourette's Syndrome Global Scale	TSGS	Harcherik et al, 1984
OC component (children)	Children's Yale-Brown Obsessive Compulsive Scale	CY-BOCS	Scahill et al, 1997
OC component (adults)	Yale-Brown Obsessive Compulsive Scale	Y-BOCS	Goodman et al, 1989
Tics	Rush Video-Based Tic Rating Scale	none	Goetz et al, 1999
Tic premonitory urges	Premonitory Urge for Tics Scale	PUTS	Woods et al, 2005
TS-related Quality of Life (in children)	Gilles de la Tourette Syndrome – Quality of Life Scale for Children and Adolescents	C&A-GTS	Su et al, 2017
TS-related Quality of Life (in adults)	Gilles de la Tourette Syndrome – Quality of Life Scale GTS-QOL	GTS-QOL	Cavanna et al, 2008

Diagnostic Confidence Index – DCI is a test whose result is a percentage of exactness of TS diagnosis. Every item is based on the presence/absence of a TS characteristic eg. coprolalia. Above 59%, diagnosis can be confirmed.

Yale Global Tic Severity Scale – YGTSS is the most used clinical scale to assess the severity of tics. It is divided into an objective part i.e. Tic Severity, and a subjective part i.e. Social Impairment. It is important to note that the two parts are equally divided in the Global Score: the impairment is as fundamental as the severity (Table 3.7). One of the objective subparts is frequency of motor and sound tics (see the example in Table 3.7).

Barbara (Table 3.7), an 8-year-old TS child, results in having a moderate syndrome in terms of severity. She has been helped by her parents in filling in the YGTSS because she is not aware of all her tics. Frequency is higher for Barbara's motor tics than for her sound tics.

Table 3.7 Adapted from the YGTSS scale of Barbara.

Frequency of motor tics	3 points/5: tics stop for 3 hours maximum a day
Frequency of sound tics	2 points/5: tics stop for 6 hours maximum a day
....	....
Total Tic Severity	34 points/50
Social Impairment	30 points/50
Global score:	64 points/100
Total Tic Severity	
+ Social Impairment	

The Social Impairment is medium because she has been having some tic-related difficulties with schoolmates.

Tourette's Syndrome Global Scale – TSGS is another scale used to assess tics and Social Impairment. It is comparable to YGTSS, but less used.

Yale-Brown Obsessive Compulsive Scale – Y-BOCS is the most used clinical scale for OC component in adults and *Children's Yale-Brown Obsessive Compulsive Scale – CY-BOCS* is the equivalent in children.

These two scales monitor the severity of symptoms during a treatment.

In Table 3.8, the CY-BOCS subscale frequency is taken as example. Kate, a 10-year-old TS child, results having a moderate OC component. Frequency is 2 points higher for her obsessions than for her compulsions.

Table 3.8 Adapted from the CY-BOCS of Kate.

Obsessions		
Frequency	1 point/4: symptoms are present for less than an hour per day	
....	....	
Total		12 points/20

Compulsions		
Frequency	2 points/4: symptoms are present from one to three hours per day	
....	....	
Total		10 points/20
TOTAL SCORE (OBSESSIONS+COMPULSIONS)		22 points/40

Rush Video-Based Tic Rating Scale is the most used tic video recording protocol. It was developed by Goetz, a renowned neurologist. It is better used at the end of the visit as the patient could lose control and show tics more likely compared with the first few moments.

The method consists of video recording a patient for 15 minutes from different perspectives and in various postures, alone or not. The patient is also shot while walking, reading and writing. If tics do not arise, caregivers will be asked to film the patient once they are back home.

Premonitory Urge for Tics Scale – PUTS is the worldwide used scale to assess patient's insight of premonitory urge of tics.

N.B. For the aforementioned scales, caregivers of sufferers with echolalia/echopraxia should be aware that the reading aloud of symptoms may induce them. Sometimes, even when the patient himself is reading them silently, these symptoms can appear.

Quality of Life assessment

The most important point of TS assessment is Quality of Life (QoL; Cavanna et al, 2013) because only a low QoL authorises treatment.

Who decides if QoL is impaired? Not one person alone; it is a combination of the following perspectives:

- the patient (including very young children i.e. from 5 years old onwards).
- caregivers (mainly parents, siblings and grandparents for children; partner, as well, in case of adults).
- clinicians (neurologists, psychiatrists, psychologists, educators, and so on).
- social entourage (teachers including special needs teachers, tutors, sport coaches for children; colleagues, heads and the workplace medical staff in case of adults).

These opinions are sometimes contradictory, for instance, regarding the intensity of the impairment. In this case, the TS clinical team needs to define the impairment of the patient by considering the following areas (see Figure 3.9):

- health: malignant tics and SIB undermine the body integrity.
- relationships: family, friends, schoolmates, teachers and colleagues.

- school activities: e.g. writing, reading, following lessons.
- work activities for adults: e.g. PC use, mobile phone use, car use.
- spare time: sports or other hobbies.

Specifically, the interference (Figure 3.9) of TS symptoms within these areas may be:

- objective: when a person is not able to perform daily tasks because of the symptoms (e.g. the repetition of the eye blinking tic doesn't allow Marco to read his book). In this case, we can call it "functional interference".
- subjective: when emotions interfere with the psychosocial wellness of the patient (e.g. Marco feels embarrassed with his schoolmates when he has the whistling tic). In this case, we talk about "Social Impairment".

Main clinical scales for the assessment of QoL in TS (Table 3.6):

1   YGTSS (see the previous paragraph), Social Impairment subpart. It is used in both children and adults.
2   Gilles de la Tourette Syndrome – Quality of Life Scale for Children and Adolescents – C&A-GTS-QOL. Scale areas: cognitive diseases, coprolalia/praxia, psychological diseases, physical diseases, OC component and activities of daily life. It is used in children and adolescents.

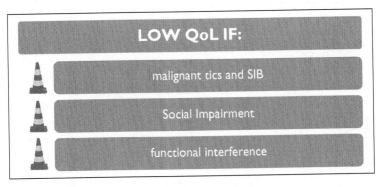

Figure 3.9 Causes of low Quality of Life in TS patients.
Credit: Cecilia Spalletti.

3 *Gilles de la Tourette Syndrome – Quality of Life Scale-GTS-QOL* is equivalent to the latter, but it is for adults.

Other tests are commonly used to assess the disorders concomitant to TS (please refer to each manual for further details):

- Schedule for Nonadaptive and Adaptive Personality – SNAP (Harlan & Clark, 1999) and Conners' ADHD Rating Scales – CRS (Conners et al 1999, Conners 2008) for ADHD.
- Child Behavior Checklist for ages 4–18 – CBCL 4-18 (Achenbach, 1991) for anxiety and depression in children.
- State-Trait Anxiety Inventory – STAI (Spielberger et al, 1970) for anxiety in adults.
- Beck Depression Inventory-second edition – BDI-II (Beck et al, 1996) for depression in adults.
- Autism Spectrum Screening Questionnaire – ASSQ (Ehlers et al, 1999) for autism spectrum disorders.
- Structured Clinical Interview for DSM-IV Axis II Personality Disorders – SCID-II (First et al, 1997) for personality disorders (adult patients).

Alert!

Results of clinical scales help to set up treatments. Families should fill in the scales forms with close attention.

Differential diagnoses

Many times, Tourette Centres' doctors visit a TS patient and make a first diagnosis or confirm the diagnosis the patient already has. In other occasions, it also happens that a differential diagnosis is needed.

A correct and clear diagnosis is the first step to hearten patients and caregivers (Figure 3.10) and to obtain their compliance.

Stereotypies versus TS (Table 3.9). Stereotypies' onset is before 2 years old whereas tics' onset is 6–7 years old. Stereotypies manifest with fixed patterns, whereas tic patterns vary. Stereotypies involve arms, hands or the entire body rather than the various tic areas.

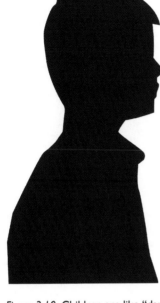

Figure 3.10 Children are like "dark shadows" until their diagnoses are defined.

Credit: Cecilia Spalletti.

Table 3.9 Differential diagnoses of TS.

Other diagnosis	Tourette syndrome features	Other diagnosis features
Stereotypies	onset: 6–7 y.o.	onset: before 2 y.o.
	varying pattern	fixed pattern (especially arms, and hands)
	non-rhythmic	rhythmic
	premonitory urge	absence of premonitory urge
	during inactivity	during activity
	often not stopped with distraction	stopped with distraction
	patient tries to stop tics	patient doesn't try to stop stereotypies
Autism spectrum disorders	normal/high IQ	low IQ
	just Social Impairment for tics	social deficiency

(continued)

Table 3.9 (continued)

Other diagnosis	Tourette syndrome features	Other diagnosis features
Dystonia	tics are often rapid and not only twisting tics	twisting and sustained posture
	tics can reduce while doing physical activity	exacerbated by physical activity
ADHD	motor and sound tics, as well	never had tics (and no familiarity for TS)
Stuttering, Dyslexia/ Dysgraphia	speech/handwriting tics, and other tics	never had tics (and no familiarity for TS)

Stereotypies are more rhythmic than tics and they are not associated with any premonitory urge. Stereotypies often manifest when the patient is absorbed in an activity such as videogames, whereas in this case tics would stop. Stereotypies can be stopped if the patient is distracted and rarely the patient tries to stop them; conversely, distraction couldn't be sufficient to stop tics, and TS patients themselves usually try to stop them.

Autism spectrum disorders versus TS (Table 3.9). Autism spectrum disorders (including also ex-Asperger Syndrome) are often accompanied by a low IQ, whereas TS is sometimes accompanied by a quite high IQ. Relationships are preserved in TS: the patient can suffer for having tics in relation with peers, but he has no social deficiency. On the contrary, social skills are approximately absent in severe autism spectrum disorder patients. OC component can be found in both pathologies, it is certainly, together with tic/stereotypies, the common element, for which a differential diagnosis is needed.

Dystonia versus TS (Table 3.9). Dystonia is a disorder in which sustained or repetitive muscle contraction result in twisting and repetitive movements or abnormal fixed postures. Tics, on the other hand, are often rapid movements, not only twisting type movements. Dystonia, unlikely tics, is often exacerbated by doing physical activity.

ADHD versus TS (Table 3.9). In order to diagnose ADHD, the patient should never have had motor or sound tics. For this reason, it is helpful to interview caregivers to collect data of the patient's childhood. Even familiarity (meaning the presence of TS or ADHD only in the relatives) may help in discriminate between the two disorders. In the case of young children (i.e. 6 years old or under), diagnosis may change from ADHD to TS if tics eventually manifest as they grow up.

Stuttering, as well as *dyslexia and dysgraphia* (Table 3.9), is often wrongly diagnosed without considering a possible Tourette diagnosis. In a TS patient, these diseases should be identified as speech/handwriting tics.

Other disorders share features with TS. One example is Rett syndrome; it can be confused with Tourette because of the similar name and because of presenting stereotypies. Rett is a severe neurologic brain syndrome, which generally affects females.

These listed differential diagnoses belong to the same neurobehavioural field. Unfortunately, doctors make wrong diagnoses, even of those belonging to other fields: a few examples are diagnoses of dermatitis and allergies. It remains imperative to develop an awareness of diagnostic criteria to avoid underdiagnosis and misdiagnosis.

Communicating the diagnosis

After the visit, the doctor has the hard task of giving a diagnosis to both the patient and the caregivers (Rivera-Navarro et al, 2009).

Box 3.1   Perception of the name "Tourette syndrome" by patients.

"Tourette syndrome" is sometimes perceived as a scary label by patients and caregivers. For this reason, many doctors diagnose "Tic Disorder" instead of TS.

Many times, it is thanks to caregivers that doctors are able to visit a patient and finally diagnose the TS condition. Together with teachers, they are often the first ones to capture the initial signs. In some cases, parents hardly react in front of the diagnosis (see also Chapter 5). It is, therefore, helpful to reassure them by telling that TS can be a transient disorder ("It decreases, or will even naturally resolve, between 18 and 30 years old"). The doctor should also explain that symptoms will wax-and-wane, therefore treatments could often be suspended (see Chapter 4).

The doctor might introduce the patient's family to other families with members having the same spectrum or of a similar age, or undergoing the same treatment. This allows them to talk about their syndrome's history, and to support each other with their own experiences.

In the event of a great emotional reaction to the unforeseen diagnosis, psychological visits could be suggested (to the patient or to their caregivers).

Prognosis

Prognosis is difficult to define, as the reader can understand from the variability of the TS symptoms presented in this chapter. Despite this, recent studies have highlighted some key points about prognosis. Predictors of increased tic severity in adulthood include higher childhood tic severity (Hassan & Cavanna, 2012) and TS familiarity (Carter et al, 1994). Furthermore, untreated comorbid psychopathologies, e.g. ADHD or OC component, is another negative prognostic factor (Hassan & Cavanna, 2012).

No prognostic tests are available currently, therefore further studies are needed to build them.

Usually the doctor chooses not to express his view about the future spectrum of the patient. A doctor can, instead, confirm with certainty the natural regression of the syndrome with the growing of the child. Unknown prognosis is another hard point for the life of a TS patient and his family as they often don't know how to organise their lives in relation to the syndrome. Fortunately, nowadays, TS patients and families can quickly consult TS associations and follow the scientific progress of TS research with the help of media.

Conclusions

TS diagnosis is not only given by tics; behavioural problems are also part of the disease and often they are the most disabling symptoms for the patient. This has led to consider TS as a neurodevelopmental disorder having behavioural traits.

TS assessment must be focused on Social Impairment, SIB and daily interference, taking into account the variability of the symptoms during childhood. Moreover, TS sufferers can be grouped in at least five subtypes depending on their manifestations.

New diagnostic and prognostic criteria are needed, including ones based on biological examinations.

Raising awareness of TS would also guarantee early and correct diagnoses.

References

Achenbach T. 1991. *Manual for the Child Behavior Checklist for Ages 4-18 (CBCL 4-18)*. Burlington, VT, USA: University Associate on Psychiatry.

American Psychiatric Association. 2013. Tic disorders. In: *Diagnostic and Statistical Manual of Mental Disorders-fifth edition; DSM-5*. Arlington, VA, USA: American Psychiatric Publishing, 81–85.

Baron-Cohen S, Scahill VL, Izaguirre J, Hornsey H, & Robertson MM. 1999. The prevalence of Gilles de la Tourette syndrome in children and adolescents with autism: A large scale study. Vol 29. *Psychological Medicine*, 1151–1159.

Beck AT, Steer RA, & Brown GK. 1996. *Beck Depression Inventory-second edition (BDI-II)*. San Antonio, TX, USA: The Psychological Corporation.

Bloch MH. 2013. Clinical courser and adult outcome in Tourette's Syndrome. In: Martino D, Leckman JF, eds. *Tourette Syndrome*. Oxford, UK: Oxford University Press, 107–120.

Bloch MH & Leckman JF. 2009. Clinical course of Tourette syndrome. Vol 67. *Journal of Psychosomatic Research*, 497–501.

Cavanna AE, Robertson MM, & Critchley HD. 2007. Schizotypal personality traits in Gilles de la Tourette syndrome. Vol 116(6). *Acta Neurologica Scandinavica*, 385–391.

Cavanna AE, Schrag A, Morley D, Orth M, Robertson MM, Joyce E, . . . , & Selai C. 2008. The Gilles de la Tourette syndrome-quality of life scale (GTS-QOL): development and validation. Vol 71(18). *Neurology*, 1410–1416.

Cavanna AE, Luoni C, Selvini C, Blangiardo R, Eddy CM, Silvestri PR, . . . , & Termine C. 2013. Disease-specific quality of life in young patients with Tourette syndrome. Vol 48(2). *Pediatric Neurology*, 111–114.

Carter AS, Pauls DL, Leckman JF, & Cohen DJ. 1994. A prospective longitudinal study of Gilles de la Tourette's syndrome. Vol 33. *Journal of the American Academy of Child & Adolescent Psychiatry*, 377–385.

Conners K, Erhardt E, & Sparrow E. 1999. *Adult ADHD Rating Scales*. North Tonawanda, NY, USA: Multi Health Systems.

Conners CK. 2008. *Conners 3rd Edition (Conners 3)*. North Tonawanda, NY, USA: Multi Health Systems.

Dell'Osso B, Marazziti D, Albert U, Pallanti S, Gambini O, Tundo A, . . . , & Porta M. 2017. Parsing the phenotype of obsessive-compulsive tic disorder (OCTD): A multidisciplinary consensus. Vol 21(2). *International Journal of Psychiatry in Clinical Practice*, 156–159.

Ehlers S, Gillberg C, & Wing L. 1999. A screening questionnaire for Asperger syndrome and other high-functioning autism spectrum disorders in school age children. Vol 29. *Journal of Autism and Developmental Disorders*, 129–141.

First MB, Gibbon M, Spitzer RL, Williams JBW, & Benjamin LS. 1997. *Structured Clinical Interview for DSM-IV Axis II Personality Disorders (SCID-II)*. Washington DC, MD, USA: American Psychiatric Press.

Erenberg G, Cruse RP, & Rothner AD. 1987. The natural history of Tourette syndrome: A follow-up study. Vol 22(3). *Annals of Neurology*, 383–385.

Freeman RD, Fast DK, Burd L, Kerbeshian J, Robertson MM, & Sandor P. 2000. An international perspective on Tourette syndrome: Selected findings from 3,500 individuals in 22 countries. Vol 42. *Developmental Medicine & Child Neurology*, 436–447.

Goetz CG, Pappert EJ, Louis ED, Raman R, & Leurgans S. 1999. Advantages of a modified scoring method for the Rush Video-Based Tic Rating Scale. Vol 14(3). *Movement Disorders*, 502–506.

Goodman WK, Price LH, Rasmussen SA, Mazure C, Fleischmann RL, Hill CL, . . . , & Charney DS. 1989. The Yale-Brown Obsessive Compulsive Scale. I: Development, use, and reliability. Vol 46(11). *Archives of General Psychiatry*, 1006–1011.

Grados MA, Mathews CA, & The Tourette Syndrome Association International Consortium for Genetics. 2008. Latent class analysis of Gilles de la Tourette syndrome using comorbidities: Clinical and genetic implications. Vol 64. *Biological Psychiatry*, 219–225.

Harcherik DF, Leckman JF, Detlor J, & Cohen DJ. 1984. A new instrument for clinical studies of Tourette's syndrome. Vol 23(2). *Journal of the American Academy of Child & Adolescent Psychiatry*, 153–160.

Harlan E & Clark LA. 1999. Short forms of the Schedule for Nonadaptive and Adaptive Personality (SNAP) for self- and collateral ratings: Development, reliability, and validity. Vol 6. *Assessment*, 131–145.

Hassan N & Cavanna AE. 2012. The prognosis of Tourette syndrome: Implications for clinical practice. Vol 27(1). *Functional Neurology*, 23–27.

Hirschtritt ME, Darrow SM, Illmann C, Osiecki L, Grados M, Sandor P, . . . , & Mathews CA. 2018. Genetic and phenotypic overlap of specific obsessive-compulsive and attention-deficit/hyperactive subtypes with Tourette syndrome. Vol 48(2). *Psychological Medicine*, 279–293.

Hollander E & Rosen J. 2000. Impulsivity. Vol 14(2 suppl 1). *Journal of Psychopharmacology*, S39–44.

Jankovic J & Kurlan R. 2011. Tourette syndrome: evolving concepts. Vol 26(6). *Movement Disorders*, 1149–1156.

Leckman JF & Cohen D. 1999. *Tourette's Syndrome. Tics, Obsessions, Compulsions, Developmental Psychopathology and Clinical Care*. New York City, NY, USA: Wiley, 24–26, 37–41.

Leckman JF, Riddle MA, Hardin MT, Ort SI, Swartz KL, Stevenson J, & Cohen DJ. 1989. The Yale Global Tic Severity Scale: Initial testing of a clinician-rated scale of severity. Vol 28. *Journal of the American Academy of Child & Adolescent Psychiatry*, 566–573.

Martino D, Chiarotti F, Buttiglione M, Cardona F, Creti R, Nardocci N, . . ., & Italian Tourette Syndrome Study Group. 2011. The relationship between group A streptococcal infections and Tourette syndrome: a study on a large service-based cohort. Vol 53(10). *Developmental Medicine & Child Neurology*, 951–957.

Martino D, Zis P, & Buttiglione M. 2015. The role of immune mechanisms in Tourette syndrome. Vol 1617. *Brain Research*, 126–143.

Mol Debes NM, Hjalgrim H, & Skov L. 2008. Limited knowledge of Tourette syndrome causes delay in diagnosis. Vol 39. *Neuropediatrics*, 101–105.

Morand-Beaulieu S, Leclerc JB, Valois P, Lavoie ME, O'Connor KP, & Gauthier B. 2017. A review of the neuropsychological dimensions of Tourette Syndrome. Vol 7(8). *Brain Science*. 106.

Müller N, Riedel M, Straube A, Günther W, Wilske B. 2000. Increased anti-streptococcal antibodies in patients with Tourette's syndrome. Vol 94. *Psychiatry Research*, 43–49.

Porta M & Sironi VA. 2017. *Il cervello irriverente*. Bari, IT, EU: Editori Laterza, 85–95.

Rivera-Navarro J, Cubo E, & Almazán J. 2009. The diagnosis of Tourette's Syndrome: Communication and impact. Vol 14(1). *Clinical Child Psychology and Psychiatry*, 13–23.

Robertson MM. 1989. The Gilles de la Tourette syndrome: The current status. Vol 154. *British Journal of Psychiatry*, 147–169.

Robertson MM, Banerjee S, Kurlan R, Cohen DJ, Leckman JF, McMahon W, . . ., van de Wetering BJ. 1999. The Tourette syndrome diagnostic confidence index: Development and clinical associations. Vol 53. *Neurology*, 2108–2112.

Robertson MM, Trimble MR, & Lees AJ. 1989. Self-injurious behaviour and the Gilles de la Tourette syndrome: A clinical study and review of the literature. Vol 19(3). *Psychological Medicine*, 611–625.

Robertson MM. 2000. Tourette syndrome, associated conditions and the complexities of treatment. Vol 123. *Brain*, 425–462.

Robertson MM. 2006. Tourette Syndrome and affective disorders: an update. Vol 61. *Journal of Psychosomatic Research*, 349–358.

Robertson MM. 2015. A personal 35 year perspective on Gilles de la Tourette syndrome: prevalence, phenomenology, comorbidities, and coexistent psychopathologies. Vol 2(1). *Lancet Psychiatry*, 68–87.

Robertson MM, Cavanna AE, & Eapen V. 2015. Gilles de la Tourette syndrome and disruptive behavior disorders: prevalence, associations, and explanation of the relationships. Vol 27(1). *Journal of Neuropsychiatry and Clinical Neurosciences*, 33–41.

Rothenberger A & Roessner V. 2013. The phenomenology of attention deficit hyperactivity disorder in Tourette Syndrome. In: Martino D & Leckman JF, eds. *Tourette Syndrome*. Oxford, UK, EU: Oxford University Press, 26–49.

Scahill L, Riddle MA, McSwiggin-Hardin M, Ort SI, King RA, Goodman WK, . . . , & Leckman JF. 1997. Children's Yale-Brown Obsessive Compulsive Scale: Reliability and validity. Vol 36(6). *Journal of the American Academy of Child & Adolescent Psychiatry*, 844–852.

Scalone L, D'Angiolella LS, Mantovani LG, Galentino R, Servello D, Dell'Osso B, . . . , & Porta M. 2017. Obsessive Compulsive Tic Disorder: Appropriate diagnosis and treatment as key elements to improve health and rationalize use of resources. Vol 14(4). *Epidemiology Biostatistics and Public Health*, e12661-9.

Spielberger CD, Gorsuch RL, & Lushene RE. 1970. *Manual for the State-Trait Anxiety Inventory*. Palo Alto, CA, USA: Consulting Psychologist Press.

Su MT, McFarlane F, Cavanna AE, Termine C, Murray I, Heidemeyer L, . . . , & Murphy T. 2017. The English Version of the Gilles de la Tourette Syndrome-Quality of Life Scale for Children and Adolescents (C&A-GTS-QOL). Vol 32(1). *Journal of Child Neurology*, 76–83.

Swedo SE, Leonard HL, Garvey M, Mittleman B, Allen AJ, Perlmutter S, Lougee L, Dow S, Zamkoff J, & Dubbert BK. 1998. Pediatric autoimmune neuropsychiatric disorders associated with streptococcal infections: Clinical description of the first 50 cases. Vol 155(2). *American Journal of Psychiatry*, 264–71.

The Tourette Syndrome Classification Study Group. 1993. Definitions and classification of tic disorders. Vol 50. *Archives of Neurology*, 1013–1016.

Trillini MO & Müller-Vahl KR. 2015. Patients with Gilles de la Tourette syndrome have widespread personality differences. Vol 228(3). *Psychiatry Research*, 765–773.

Woods DW, Piacentini J, Himle MB, & Chang S. 2005. Premonitory Urge for Tics Scale (PUTS): Initial psychometric results and examination of the premonitory urge phenomenon in youths with Tic disorders. Vol 26(6). *Journal of Developmental & Behavioral Pediatrics*, 397–403.

World Health Organization (WHO). 2003. Multiaxial classification of child and adolescent psychiatric disorders. In: *International Statistical Classification of Diseases and Related Health Problems-tenth revision (ICD-10)*. Cambridge, UK, EU: Cambridge University Press, 221–223.

Wright A, Rickards H, & Cavanna AE. 2012. Impulse-control disorders in Gilles de la Tourette syndrome. Vol 24(1). *The Journal of Neuropsychiatry and Clinical Neurosciences*, 6-27.

Zanaboni Dina C, Bona AR, Zekaj E, Servello D, & Porta M. 2016. Handwriting tics in Tourette's syndrome: A single center study. Vol 7. *Front Psychiatry*, 15.

Chapter 4

Therapy for Tourette syndrome*

Summary

The main aim of TS therapy is to improve Quality of Life (QoL) for the sufferer. In order to reach this goal, one or more treatments can be tailored on a case by case basis. It must be stressed that a major problem regarding therapy is the low compliance of TS patients and caregivers, which needs to be stimulated by clinicians.

The first step to be considered is Habit Reversal Training (HRT), a method of Cognitive Behavioural Therapy (CBT) for the management of tics in both children and adults. The training helps the patient to develop awareness of the TS symptoms, and it promotes an alternative response, i.e. "a new habit" in contrast with a target tic. The second step to be considered is pharmacological therapy (acting on the different neurotransmitters responsible for TS symptoms): mainly antipsychotics and antidepressants, but also antihypertensives, antibiotics and other agents.

The two mini-invasive treatments are botulinum toxin and, extremely rarely, Deep Brain Stimulation, that are only used in adult severe refractory cases.

Introduction

Alert!

Treatments are only for TS patients with significant impaired QoL.

---

* In collaboration with Matteo Briguglio and Alberto Riccardo Bona

TS can be treated. This is good news! Many patients and caregivers often arrive to Tourette Centres with confused ideas about treatment options. A good clinician should, therefore, introduce the patient (and caregivers) to the different possibilities of treatments (Table 4.1). Treatment(s) choice is linked to TS severity (see Figure 4.1). For this reason, the different options are reported here, considering treatments from the least severe to the most severe form of TS. The therapeutic algorithm follows this order: observation, psychoeducation, Cognitive Behavioural Therapy (CBT) including Habit Reversal Training (HRT) and other techniques. For more severe forms of TS, the therapeutic options are: pharmacological treatments, botulinum toxin and, rarely, Deep Brain Stimulation (DBS).

Furthermore, patients should be told that treatments are *combinable* and *variable* considering the course of the syndrome (the scientific word for this concept is "add-on treatment"). When referring to the word "combinable", it means a combination of more than one treatment. According to the spectrum of each patient (cf. Chapter 3), the TS team opts for a single or for a combination of treatments. For instance, a patient with a medium to severe spectrum could benefit from HRT+pharmacological treatment; whereas a very simple spectrum patient could benefit from psychoeducation alone.

On the other hand, the variability ("variable") of the spectrum during the course of the syndrome (cf. Chapter 3) requires a variability in the treatment. For example, Paul can be treated with mild medications only, when he is 6 years old and he has just slight tics; then, when he is a teenager and his spectrum extends to the psychopathological sphere, he can be treated with both HRT and pharmacological treatments. When he grows up and his symptoms reduce, he can stop treatments.

Table 4.1 Brief description of main TS treatments.

Brief description of TS treatments	
Observation	Monitoring symptoms with the help of a diary given by the doctor
Psychoeducation	Sessions about the functioning of the syndrome, held by a psychologist
CBT (including HRT)	Sessions focused on the patient's own syndrome, held by a psychotherapist
Pharmacological treatments	Drugs to treat TS symptoms
Other (exceptional) treatments	Injections and other medical techniques

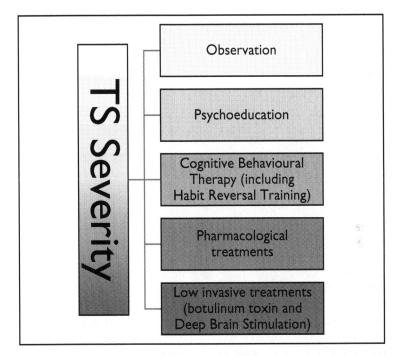

Figure 4.1 TS treatments according to the patient's severity. Treatments may be combined.

Credit: Cecilia Spalletti.

Treatment steps should also be *consequential* by following the sequence of Figure 4.1. This indicates that a patient should be treated with a step only after having be treated with the previous ones. For example, Martha can't be treated directly with DBS without a trial of observation, psychoeducation, CBT and medications. Exceptions are practicable when considering case-by-case conditions.

TS International Guidelines and a local Ethical Committee guide treatment choice. The most recent international treatment guidelines are:

- *UK* (Cavanna et al, 2011).
- *Europe* (Roessner et al, 2011a; Cath et al, 2011 ; Roessner et al, 2011b; Verdellen et al, 2001; Müller-Vahl et al, 2011).
- *Canada* (Sandor & Carrol, 2012; Pringsheim et al, 2012; Steeves et al, 2012).

An Ethical Committee is an authority group, including clinicians, lawyers and churchmen, within hospitals. It has a decisional role with the goal of protecting the rights, safety and well-being of patients.

Observation and psychoeducation

The first clinical step to be considered for a TS patient is a period of observation, after the diagnosis or the presumed diagnosis. Symptoms need to be present for a year to make the diagnosis (cf. Chapter 3). The observation period requires a diary – completed by the patient or by the caregiver – to follow the trend of symptoms. The diary is also a proper technique in the sense that it reduces the frequency or intensity of symptoms recorded (see Table 4.3; Verdellen et al, 2011). For this reason, observation can be considered a first form of treatment. It is also helpful to reassure patients and caregivers about their TS-related fears. The period of observation can be 9–11 months long as a maximum. A second therapeutic step may then be necessary. It all depends on the level of Social Impairment of the patient. If the level is low and there are no SIB nor malignant tics nor functional interference, the observation period may be concluded with no other intervention; otherwise, the TS team would opt for the best treatment option.

The second clinical step to consider, when talking about TS treatments, is psychoeducation. Psychoeducation means that patients and caregivers attend sessions to learn about the functioning of the

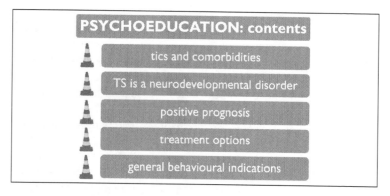

Figure 4.2 Psychoeducation in TS: principal contents.
Credit: Cecilia Spalletti.

syndrome (Verdellen et al, 2011; cf. Figure 4.2). Sessions can consist of one or more, and they are both informative (tics, comorbidities, TS as a neurodevelopmental disorder, positive prognosis, treatment options) and formative (behavioural indications). Clinicians will indeed give the patients and the caregivers some practical suggestions. For instance, the patient could modify his bedtime in order to reduce tics and OC component, which usually increase in the evening. The behavioural indications are general prompts suitable for every TS person, whereas if a patient needs his own consultation a Habit Reversal Training or other type of intervention should be considered.

Habit Reversal Training

Since the 1970s, Habit Reversal Training (HRT; Azrin & Nunn, 1973) is the gold standard of psychotherapy for TS (McGuire et al, 2015). HRT reduces up to 37.5% of tics (Dutta & Cavanna, 2013).

This method originates from Cognitive Behavioural Therapy (CBT; cf. Table 4.1). CBT is an evidence-based practice; it works on the change of dysfunctional cognitive and behavioural patterns, and consequently on the emotional regulation.

CBT can be considered a "fast" psychotherapy because of the homework involved. In fact, the patient trains not only during the sessions but also every day thanks to homework. In this way, the patient will quickly become independent from the therapist as they can continue to work by themselves.

Rationale

In this chapter, the authors discuss a model of HRT+other CBT techniques as many clinicians (Woods et al, 2008; Piacentini et al, 2010; CZD) have experienced higher efficacy in TS when compared with HRT only.

In HRT the tic is considered as a habit, and therefore, it can be modified.

Session by session, the tic will be acknowledged and substituted with another movement (see Figure 4.3). By substituting it, the premonitory urge will be satisfied, and the necessity of the tic will vanish. Before this final and specific exercise though, many other cognitive and behavioural techniques are adopted to reduce – both objectively (e.g. tic frequency) and subjectively (Social Impairment) – the tic. In fact, the goal of the intervention is to improve QoL.

At first, the focus is on the causes of tic increase. Later, when it is impossible or insufficient to modify the cause, the intervention should modify the tic habit. N.B. tics are mainly neurological, but psychological components can increase them. CBT works on the psychological causes of tic increase, when there are some or, when psychological causes are absent, directly on the neurological basis of tics.

Participants

HRT is suitable for non-severe TS children and adults, starting from 6 years of age (see Figure 4.3).

Regarding the required cognitive abilities, it would be better to offer HRT to patients with very low or absent cognitive deficits. In case of medium deficits i.e. patients with IQ≈85, HRT can be done with a simplified method. Additionally, the authors speculate that the more patients are aware of their own tics and can reproduce them, the more they can benefit from the training itself.

Once the HRT has started (in case of minors), at least one parent should be present at the sessions. In this way, parents can help the patient with the homework. Furthermore, caregivers could be involved in the symptoms of the patient (cf. Chapter 3) and, as a consequence, it would be helpful to share their point of view.

When the patient can't follow a HRT programme (cf. Figure 4.3), Parent Training treatment becomes an option. "Parent Training" means that the parents of a patient are involved in a specific-disease training to help their child.

Parent Training in TS (cf. Table 4.2) may be a therapeutic choice in the following cases:

- The child is following a HRT program, but the parents need a separate consultation.
- The sufferer's parents have different parenting styles.

Table 4.2 Psychological interventions in TS: n° and type of participants.

Number of participants	Type of participants	Name of the intervention
Minimum 1 person	Patient (and caregivers)	HRT
2 people	Parents	Parent Training
≥2 people	Group of patients	Self-help group

- The sufferer's parents highlight tics, and therefore provoke a tic increase.
- The child is too young or not sufficiently motivated for a HRT program (see paragraph "Motivation").
- The child's cognitive level is not appropriate for a HRT programme.

Parent Training consists in analysing symptomatic episodes with the aim of promoting new parents' cognitive-behavioural patterns.

HRT can't be done in a group as homework is adapted for each patient's needs. Vice versa, group can be employed for psychoeducation (cf. paragraph, "Observation and psychoeducation") or for self-help groups (Table 4.2). Self-help groups are groups of people, who share a problem, in this case TS. N.B. TS self-help groups should be guided by an expert, at least.

Motivation

What is mandatory in HRT is the motivation of the patients in attending sessions regularly and in doing homework (see also paragraph, "Compliance"). For this reason, every session closes with a shared decision on homework for the next session. In cases where the motivation is not high enough, the therapist can decide to work on increasing motivation before starting HRT.

The following example is used to understand the importance of the issue. Paul is a patient that socially suffers from his tics (Social Impairment scoring 40 out of 50, given by his tic-related school absences): a treatment is, in his case, strictly required. The problem is that his motivation is low and he cannot take drugs because of his general medical condition. The therapist would indeed decide to work on Paul's motivation.

In non-severe cases, the therapist could also wait for the person's motivation to increase; motivation often increases because of symptoms becoming more severe, or because of the individual growth and maturity.

Timing

Each session lasts 45 minutes but some psychotherapists prefer to conclude in 60 minutes. According to the author (CZD) it would be better to evaluate each individual case. As an example, for a TS patient with ADHD, 60 minutes would be better as many pauses are necessary to keep the patient focused. It could be that another TS+ADHD patient can't be active for more than 45 minutes (breaks included).

Sessions are weekly, every 10 days at maximum. While reaching the goals, sessions gradually become less frequent (e.g. one every other week, and then one every 20 days, and so on).

Between sessions, the patient will complete homework: usually Monday to Friday for roughly five minutes a day.

Setting

CBT is a face-to-face therapy. The therapist meets the patient and the caregiver(s) in a clinical room. A table and chairs are the only necessities as the patient, together with the therapist, has to write down homework. If children are involved in the session, a few games should be available in the room to facilitate the training.

Internet-based sessions have been used in recent times instead of face-to-face ones (Holmberg & Kähkönen, 2011), but only in specific and rare cases. They are generally offered to patients living far away from the TS therapist's study (nowadays, TS specialists are few). Of course, the patient must be selected before starting with Internet-based therapy. Patients with no cognitive deficits and no severe TS psychopathologies can be good candidates. In other cases, Internet-based therapy can't be offered as it would be insufficient, for lack of real-life interaction. For instance, a

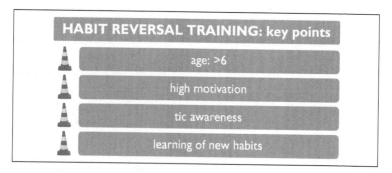

Figure 4.3 Key points of HRT.
Credit: Cecilia Spalletti.

patient with social anxiety (Clark & Wells, 1995) is not suitable for this type of therapy as it would be better for them to work on social skills (including non-verbal communication) in the therapist's office.

Aim of each session

A model of HRT+other CBT techniques is described: 10 sessions follow as a therapeutic program for a singular tic. After these, the patient can choose between continuing by themselves as they will already be familiar with the method, or continuing with the therapist. The aim of the therapy is the autonomy of the patient: as soon as possible the therapist should suggest reducing the frequency of sessions or concluding the training.

Session 1

At first, the therapist and the patient introduce themselves and the patient is asked about their expectations of the treatment. Afterwards the therapist shortly illustrates the CBT paradigm and underlines the importance of motivation and of homework.

Tics are usually of more than one type. And the target tic – the chosen tic to work on – is the one from which the person suffers the most. Only in case of SIB or malignant tics, is the patient encouraged to choose between them. Often, the most disabling tic for the patient is not the most annoying one for the caregivers (i.e. loud sound tics).

At this point, the sufferer is asked to name the target tic. Often patients identify themselves with the symptoms, whereas if they start to see tics as something external (even with a funny name), they can more easily accept the syndrome, and treat it successfully.

A diary is developed with the patient, having the premonitory urge/tic description written in chronological order (i.e. sensations/movements in order of their appearance) and as accurate as possible (see Table 4.3) to stimulate the patient's awareness (cf. Figure 4.3). This is usually the first homework.

John (Table 4.3) choses "Ugly" (blinking) as his target tic. Maximum values of "Ugly" are reached during the evening. John will soon notice that a diary is a helpful instrument to improve his awareness about tics (Figure 4.3) and to reduce them!

Table 4.3 Example of John's tic description and diary.

Tic name: "UGLY"

Premonitory urge: left eye itch.

Tic description: double left eye blinking, then right eye blinking.

	Monday	Tuesday	Wednesday	Thursday	Friday
Afternoon (1st half)	XX			X	XX
Afternoon (2nd half)		XX	X		
Evening	XXX				XXX

N.B. X/XX/XXX correspond to a specific legend of frequency and/or intensity.

Session 2

Homework is first checked and commented on. If the case of unfinished homework, a motivation analysis is needed before continuing the programme.

The patient will be then reminded of the nature of tics. Tics have a neurodevelopmental origin, but they increase because of triggers caused by intense emotions, periods of the day, types of activity and physical conditions.

Frequent triggers for tics are:

- night time
- watching TV
- tiredness/sleepiness
- stress and anxiety
- talking about it
- relaxation after stress
- boredom
- doing school homework
- meal time
- seating position
- unexpected changes
- in the car
- excitement

The patient is explained to that all emotions are useful to monitor one's status and change something when necessary. Through the "emotion alphabetisation", the therapist discusses with the patient about each emotion, related body reactions and verbal expressions.

At the end of the session, the patient will be assigned the homework of noting triggers in his diary in case of "XXX", that is when tic frequency/intensity increases (see Table 4.3).

Session 3

At the beginning, diary and the main triggers of the week are discussed. The diary is revised and the patient is prepared for a deeper analysis of triggers to be done as homework for the following session.

Then, a relaxation technique (Azrin & Peterson, 1988; Peterson & Azrin, 1992) is chosen according to the preference of the patient.

The diaphragmatic breathing is commonly used in TS as a relaxation technique (cf. Table 4.4). During tics many patients have an altered breath. The therapist will therefore accompany the sufferer to pay attention to his own breath, and she will explain the alteration of breathing in relation with emotions (Figure 4.4). She will then illustrate the diaphragmatic breathing techniques to the sufferer, and the therapist and sufferer will try it together. N.B. Experiencing exercises with the therapist gives self-confidence to the patient, who then has to train by himself at home.

The diaphragmatic breathing is realised by comparing the number of the person's normal breathing cycles (one cycle comprehends inhaling and exhaling) with the number of the person's diaphragmatic breathing cycles in the same period of time. A reasonable number of cycles to reach with the diaphragmatic breathing is 10 per minute.

The therapist will suggest being in a comfortable position to do this homework, away from distractions. It is better to use both mouth and nose to breathe. Once the patient inhales, the belly will inflate, and the belly will deflate while the patient will exhale.

Table 4.4 Relaxation techniques and references.

Relaxation technique	R
diaphragmatic breathing	Lum, 1977
progressive muscular relaxation	Jacobson, 1938; Bernstein and Borkovec, 1973

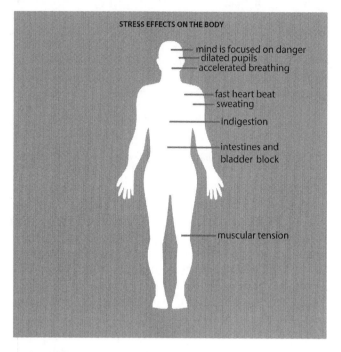

Figure 4.4 Effects of stress on the body.
Credit: Cecilia Spalletti.

The patient will be recommended to use the exercise in case of negative emotions or thoughts, or in case of tic or compulsions, or every time he feels that he can benefit from it.

The progressive muscular relaxation (cf. Table 4.4) is another relaxation technique that can be used for TS patients. This technique is specifically concentrated on a body area that could be the same of the target tic. For example (cf. Figure 4.5), Monica has a hand tic and the therapist shows her the progressive muscular relaxation on hands.

This exercise helps the patient to notice the difference between tension and relaxation of a specific body part (N.B. there are exercises focusing on every part of the body). During the manifestation of tics, patients usually tense the body area involved in the tic and, in some occasions, other body areas at the same time (Figure 4.4).

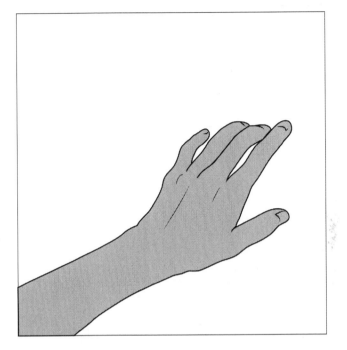

Figure 4.5 Hand progressive muscular relaxation of Monica, a TS teenager.
Credit: Cecilia Spalletti.

In the example (Figure 4.5), Monica is asked to compare her body sensations of tension/relaxation while lifting her hand from a table. Levels of tension (e.g. 0 to 3) of every part of her body will be asked before and after the hand movement (Table 4.5), consequently she is able to recognise how body tension gradually modifies through her movement. Usually level of tension decreases after it (Table 4.5). And even if the exercise is focused on the hand, a relaxation can be induced in every part of the body (see the decrease of leg tension in Table 4.5).

The technique also aims to relax the patient. The relaxation is given by the attention being focused only on a slow movement, and by the soft voice used by the therapist to guide the patient. As a result, the person is distracted from tics and negative thoughts, and reaches a relaxation state.

Homework for next session should be to continue the diary (marking triggers), and in addition, to practise a relaxation technique at least twice a week.

Table 4.5 Progressive muscular relaxation: tension before and after the exercise.

Part of the body	Tension 0–3 before the exercise	Tension 0–3 after the exercise
Hands	2	1
Legs	1	0
…	…	…

Session 4

After checking homework, the symptoms of the week are analysed with the ABC technique (also called "functional analysis"; Hanley et al, 2003; Piacentini et al, 2010). This technique consists for the patient in writing what happens, how they feel, how they behave, what they think before (A), during (B) and after the symptom (C). Finally, the patient writes their reflections on the situation, together with alternatives in thinking or behaviour.

Table 4.6 shows an analysis of a tic episode. At first, antecedents (date, time of the day, situation) are described: Peter decides to play instead of studying. Then, the problematic column describes dysfunctional emotions (0 to 10 of intensity), behaviours (tics and

Table 4.6 ABC analysis of a tic episode.

A (antecedents)	B (problem)	C (consequences)	Reflections & alternatives
1th October 2017 9 pm Tomorrow Peter has an oral Maths test at school. Peter didn't study till night as he would rather play videogames with his friend Paul.	Sniffing tic while studying at night. Anxiety 8/10 "I don't have enough time to study". Bad studying.	Peter got a bad mark in the test. Regret 7/10 "Now I have to do another oral test to get a good mark".	I should have studied before playing because at night I am too tired and anxious to prepare a test. Anxiety makes my tics worse. Next time I will study at first, then – if I still have spare time – I will play with Paul.

Table 4.7 Elettra's catch of tic "boring".

Date, time, activity	Before tic	During tic	After tic	Therapist/ caregiver
3rd March 2017, 4 pm, TV	XX		XXX	XXX
5th March 2017, 8 pm, school homework	XXX	XXXX	X	
7th March 2017, 6 pm, video games	XXX	XX		

others) and thoughts (in brackets): Peter feels anxious, tries to study with scarce success and has many tics. In the third column, consequences are described: Peter finally got a bad mark, he regrets his bad decision and has to prepare for another test. In the fourth column, reflections and alternatives are reported: Peter understands that study should be his priority, even to reduce tics. Many other ABCs may be done during the training.

"Tic catch exercise" (Table 4.7) is the next exercise that aims to gradually make the patient able to signal the tic arrival.

The patient has to say "tic" as soon as she recognises the tic arrival in a fixed period of time, e.g. 10 minutes. She has to note down the time she starts the exercise and the activity she has chosen to do during it (cf. Table 4.7). A daily activity should be done during the exercise to make it more realistic. The patient should start to do the tic catch with simple activities (e.g. talking with mom about the school day), to then escalate to more difficult ones (e.g. reading a book).

In the example, every time Elettra is able to say "tic" before the tic arrival, she will put a "X" in the first column; when saying "tic" during the tic manifestation, she will put a "X" in the second column. Finally, if she says "tic" after the tic manifestation, she will put a "X" in the third column, in case she doesn't recognise the tic arrival, the therapist/caregiver will say "tic", putting a "X" in the fourth column.

The goal of the tic catch is to gradually collect more and more first column's "X", meaning the person will be able to recognise the tic before its arrival. This step is mandatory to finally substitute the specific tic with an alternative response (cf. session number 6).

Usually the tic catch homework is done 3 times a week by the patient with the help of the caregiver. Tic catches, diary, ABCs and relaxation techniques are assigned as homework.

Session 5

In this session, the principal aim is to train the tic catch. Meanwhile, the diary is constantly analysed through ABCs. Therefore, tic catches made at home are compared with tic catches made during the current session with the therapist. Finally, homework is assigned, including diary, relaxation techniques, ABCs when needed, and other tic catch practising to improve the technique.

Session 6

In session number 6, the patient learns to substitute the tic with an alternative response. Here it follows a list of alternative response of tics (Table 4.8). It is fundamental to choose an alternative response to be more socially acceptable than the tic itself, and to disable the tic manifestation. Actually, the two movements need to use antagonist muscles.

The TS person should try repeatedly the exercise to limit the new movement as subtle as possible even still substituting the tic.

Table 4.8 Examples of tics and their alternative response.

Tic	Alternative response
Eyes blinking	Opening eyes wide
Shoulders lifting	Keeping elbows along the hips
Mouth opening	Lips squeezing
Nose wrinkling	Nose lengthening
Fingers cracking	Place your hands on knees and squeeze tightly
Whistling	Diaphragmatic breathing

Table 4.9 James' tic substitution/tic catch.

Alternative response of "black tic" (blinking): opening eyes wide.

Date, time, situation	Before tic	During tic	After tic	Therapist/ caregiver
10th June 2017, 2 pm, TV	√√		X	
12th June 2017, 7 pm, school homework	√	XX		
14th June 2017, 5 pm, video games	√√√		X	

A subtle alternative response is preferable because less muscle fatigue is needed, and because it can be less visible when in public.

James (Table 4.9) tries to substitute his blinking tic with the alternative response (i.e. opening eyes wide). When he succeeds in the substitution, he will put a "√" in the first column, otherwise he will follow the same rules as for the tic catch.

N.B. The alternative response should be activated once the patient recognises the tic arrival (i.e. the premonitory urge) and it should be retained until the premonitory urge stops.

In this phase, the patient tries the substitution only during the exercise (cf. Table 4.9). From session number 7 he will try it during daily activities, as well. In doing so, he will gradually assume the substitution as new habit.

Homework for the next session is: diary, relaxation techniques, ABCs if needed and tic catches/substitutions exercises.

Session 7

Once the patient is able to substitute the tic during the exercise, they are ready to do it in their daily life. After the homework check, the therapist and the patient prepare a subjective hierarchy of more and more difficult situations (see Table 4.10), which should be gradually employed in the current session and in sessions numbers 8 and 9. The patient experiments a short period of time (e.g. 15 minutes) of tic substitution during the hierarchy of life situations, starting from the first ones.

The tic substitution in daily life, together with the diary and relaxation techniques are assigned as homework for the next session. At this point, usually typical ABCs are solved, and therefore they are no more assigned.

Table 4.10 Example of hierarchy of situations to face with the alternative response.

Level of difficulty of the situations (from the easiest to the most difficult)	Situations for the application of the alternative response to the tic
1.	During meals
2.	In the classroom
3.	While watching TV
4.	When I'm bored
5.	During homework
6.	With John

Session 8 and 9

Homework is checked and discussed. The treatment continues with the application of the substitution to different situations of the hierarchy, from situations of medium difficulty to the most difficult ones. Thanks to this practice, the patient gradually becomes autonomous from the therapist.

Homework is updated for the last session, at this point the patient is able to decide by himself for his own homework.

Session 10

Homework is checked and the patient should be able to continue on his own with upkeep homework. The follow-up sessions are defined and adapted case by case; they are usually less and less frequent (e.g. after 2 weeks, after 3 weeks, after a month, after 45 days).

In the course of HRT and in the follow-up sessions, an assessment should be repeated – and compared with the baseline assessment – to define HRT therapeutic effects.

Three false beliefs about CBT in TS:

1   tic suppression increases tics
2   tic substitution is a new tic
3   by focusing on one tic the others worsen

N.B. Here, we have presented a session-by-session description of techniques to use for tics. During sessions, techniques are adapted to the possible psychopathologies of the patient e.g. OCB.

In the following paragraph, we introduce some extra CBT techniques to use in case of these pathologies.

Other techniques of Cognitive Behavioural approach

HRT mostly treats tics, additional techniques from CBT are needed for the other TS diseases.

- When considering *anxiety* in TS, a specific psychoeducation is needed as first step. The patient should know that anxiety is a normal emotion, its primordial aim is to protect ourselves from dangers. There are two ways in which anxiety protects us thanks to the so-called "fight-or-flight" response (Cannon, 1929; Figure 4.6): attack or escape. If a person can cope with danger, the fight response will be activated. For example, if a person finds some ants at home, he will kill them.

  On the opposite, when someone can't cope with it, the flight response will be activated. For example, if a person winds up in front of a lion, he will escape.

  Anxiety becomes a disorder when the "fight-or-flight" response is activated too early in front of a situation, which is interpreted as a danger by the person, but objectively it is not. For example, Rose can feel anxiety in front of pigeons and escape from them.

  After psychoeducation, the psychotherapy pathway may be focused on anxiety issues. Relaxation techniques, diaries, ABC analysis of anxiety episodes, and gradual exposure to the anxious stimulus may all be useful techniques.

- After psychoeducation, in order to treat *depression* in TS, the therapy could include behavioural tasks (e.g. to start a specific hobby once a week), the ABC analysis of depression's episodes,

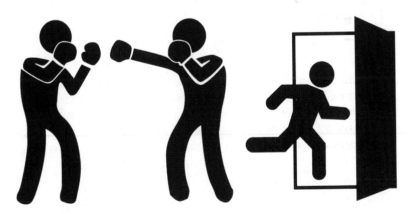

Figure 4.6 Fight-or-flight response to anxiety (Cannon, 1929).
Credit: Cecilia Spalletti.

self-esteem homework and other techniques. The authors prefer to not to discuss the topic further as it requires an in-depth section.

- *OC component* is another prevalent issue in TS. At first, it may be treated with psychoeducation, it then mainly requires an ABC analysis of the OC episodes together with the technique named "Exposure and Response Prevention" (ERP) (Verdellen et al, 2011; cf. Chapter 9). This is a gradual exposure to the obsession which usually causes the compulsion; it is sometimes used for tics too (Verdellen et al, 2011). Relaxation techniques are useful to prepare the different steps of exposure.

- *ADHD* in TS is often treated with psychoeducation, and Parent Training (cf. Subpar. "Participants"). In the Parent Training for ADHD, parents are advised how to behave to reduce symptoms. Token economy (Verdellen et al, 2011; Chapter 5 and Chapter 6) is one of the best CBT techniques to treat ADHD, together with an accurate ABC analysis of the symptomatic episodes. Token economy is a reinforcement technique in which tokens are won when the child behaves correctly. A sum of tokens for a specific period of time is rewarded with a prize. For example, John's effort in completing his CBT homework for 10 days may be rewarded with John's favourite movie.

Pharmacological treatments

Medication choice is made by the TS team based on the patient's clinical spectrum. Each symptom may require a specific drug. N.B. therapy follows the spectrum's variations.

The main goal of drug therapy, as for other TS therapies, is to reduce Social Impairment, and not to "simply" reduce/remove tics and other symptoms. Side effects must be monitored: they can't be allowed to become worse than tics! Availability of drugs and authorisation have to be carefully considered also (see paragraph "Drug-related legal/economic issues").

Treatments are "combinable" and "variable" (see paragraph, "Introduction to a variety of treatments"). This means that treatments can be associated (e.g. HRT+drugs) and changed during the course of TS.

Usually, at the beginning of the treatment, frequent control visits are needed (around every 7 to 15 days). After an initial period of time, when the clinical situation is stable, fewer visits are necessary (around 4 to 5 visits a year). In the case of children, more visits and drug trials are usually offered. During the optimisation of the drug therapy, a weekly symptom-by-symptom diary has to be completed by the patient or the caregiver.

N.B. Every change within the medication prescription must be made in person with the clinician. The law punishes those who break this safety rule.

Medical treatment is mostly based on the use of "neuromedications" to modulate the various neurotransmitters (cf. Chapter 2), or other drugs acting in different ways. According to the authors' clinical experience, TS families rarely accept the use of these drugs in their children, complicating the treatment (see paragraph, "Compliance"). Compared with other neurodevelopmental diseases, medications in TS are usually given at low dosages.

Common treatments (the class of drugs are named between dashes in the following list) in TS (cf. Roessner et al, 2011b):

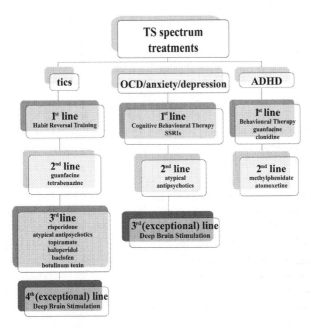

Figure 4.7 TS treatments' algorithm (Porta & Zanaboni Dina, modified from Jankovic & Kurlan, 2011).

SSRIs= Selective Serotonin Reuptake Inhibitors.

Credit: Cecilia Spalletti.

- *haloperidol* – typical antipsychotic – is the first most used drug in adult TS (Robertson, 2000) with a therapeutic effect of 78–91% on tics (Sandor et al, 1990). Despite its frequent side effects, it is also the only authorised drug for children with TS.
- *clonidine* – antihypertensive – is effective in around 50-70% of TS+ADHD cases (Cohen et al, 1980). *Guanfacine* – antihypertensive – has a similar function of clonidine, but with fewer side effects (see Figure 4.7).
- *pimozide* – typical antipsychotic – is one of the most used drug in TS (Sallee et al, 1997); pimozide, similarly to *fluphenazine* (Borison et al, 1983) – typical antipsychotic – has fewer long-term side effects if compared with haloperidol.
- *risperidone* – atypical antypsychotics – reduces TS symptoms in 40–70% of clinical cases, with low side effects (Bruun & Budman, 1996). It is a first-choice treatment for tics according to the European Guidelines (Roessner, 2011b).
- *aripiprazole, quetiapine, ziprasidone, tiapride* and *sulpiride* are atypical antipsychotics – D2 blockers (i.e. active on a specific dopamine receptor). They are mostly effective on tics and they show low side effects. For this reason, Eddy et al (2011), Roessner et al (2011b) and Singer (2010) recommend their use as first line. Authors (MP & CZD) recommend their use as second line (see Figure 4.7). Tiapride and sulpiride are used in Europe; in the USA they are not authorised.
- *tetrabenazine* – monoamine depletors – is suitable for refractory patients to neuroleptics; no severe side effects are usually experienced with this medication.
- *fluoxetine, fluvoxamine, sertraline* and *citalopram* – SSRIs, namely Selective Serotonin Reuptake Inhibitors i.e. a type of antidepressant drugs (cf. Figure 4.7) – are commonly employed to treat the OC component in TS.
- *clomipramine* and *amitriptyline* – tricyclic antidepressants – can be used by themselves or in association with SSRIs to treat the OC component.
- *amoxicillin, diaminocillina* – antibiotics – are mostly used in the case of active streptococcal infections.
- *nicotine* patches are effective in association with haloperidol: they enhance haloperidol's effect.
- *topiramate* – anticonvulsant – is a 3rd line medication for tics.
- *baclofen* – central nervous system depressant – is another 3rd line medication for tics.

- *methylphenidate* – stimulant – is a 2nd line medication for ADHD in TS (see Figure 4.7).
- *atomoxetine* – norepinephrine reuptake inhibitor – is another 2nd line medication for ADHD in TS (see Figure 4.7).
- *clonazepam* – benzodiazepine – is a medication for tics.
- *cortisone* – corticosteroid – is useful to regulate the immune system, responsible of TS symptoms.
- *paliperidone* – atypical antipsychotic – is more rarely used in TS.
- *cannabis* – cannabinoid – has a recent and controversial use in TS.

N.B. Cannabis' use in TS leads to severe social consequences, including drug dealing, or other medical issues such as substance abuse. Furthermore, the typical poor compliance of TS patients (see paragraph, "Compliance") plays a negative role in the management of cannabis prescription. For all these reasons, cannabis should be used only in refractory and severe patients; clinicians have to constantly verify patients' compliance.

Alert!

Medications could cause side effects.

Side effects of the listed medications may manifest in 80% of cases (Chappel et al, 1995). N.B. Side effects are, in general, temporary and they stop with drug adjustment/interruption. The main ones are:

- drowsiness.
- increased appetite.
- galactorrhea (i.e. flow of milk from the breast, unassociated with childbirth or nursing) and amenorrhea (i.e. abnormal absence of menstrual period). They are both caused by hyperprolactinemia (i.e. a hormonal dysfunction).
- extrapyramidal symptoms (i.e. drug-induced movement disorders), such as akathisia (i.e. restlessness), tardive dyskinesia (i.e. involuntary repetitive body movement), oculogyric crisis (i.e. upward deviation of the eyes), tremors, bradykinesia (i.e. slowness of movements).

- anxiety.
- depression and other mood diseases.
- aggression.
- lack of attention.
- electrocardiogram alterations, e.g. altered QT interval (the QT interval is the measure of a specific period of time in the heart's electrical cycle).
- insomnia.
- nausea and vomiting.
- hypertension.
- hypotension and hypothermia. These are rare, but they can be severe in the so-called neuroleptic malignant syndrome.
- creativity reduction.

This information about drugs has been collected from the main current guidelines about treatments in TS on behalf of the "European Clinical Guidelines for Tourette syndrome and other tic disorders (Roessner et al, 2011b)" and of the Cochrane Reviews.

Drug-related legal/economic issues

The process of getting a TS diagnosis takes more than five years (cf. Chapter 3) with a huge use of economic, health and social resources. Once the diagnostic-therapeutic pathway has been taken, two major legal/economic drug-related issues need to be mentioned:

1 *Off-label*

Many of the previously listed drugs are off-label for TS. They can be scientifically approved for TS in other countries (and not where the patient lives). In this case, the TS team has to:

- ask families to sign an informed consent as approval for the drug prescription. N.B. minors' consent is also required in many countries.
- equip families with the current TS International Guidelines, together with an appropriate explanation.

Two further points concerning off-labelled drugs:

- TS families may have problems finding it at drugstores.

o   non-TS-specialists usually don't prescribe off-label drugs because of poor experience with TS patients. On the other hand, there is still no official licence to be a TS specialist.

In the absence of scientific approval for the use of a drug in TS, the following steps are mandatory:

o   a scientific trial.
o   approval by the Ethical Committee (cf. paragraph, "Introduction") and the family.

2   *Refund*
Many TS drugs are not refundable by the National Health System. Even private insurance doesn't guarantee refunds for TS visits and treatments because of the psychopathological features of the syndrome (Jankovic and Kurlan, 2011). Because of these economic reasons, patients may have to dismiss their treatments, thus damaging their own health and, as a result, society.

Medication in TS: final considerations

Pharmacotherapy in TS is as complex as TS spectrum (cf. Chapter 3). Drug treatment is given only to patients with an impairment for two reasons: a) side effects, and b) TS drugs are symptomatic (i.e. not "curative"). Being symptomatic, drugs are used long-term, but mostly in the worsening periods (see "bouts" in Chapter 3); in the other periods, they are reduced/interrupted.

The wax-and-waning of natural TS history, the variations of the symptomatology, psychosocial factors and the controllability of symptoms by the patient complicate the understanding of drugs' therapeutic results. In some cases, tics' natural ups and downs could be confused with positive or negative therapeutic results. In order to verify the reason of the spectrum change, some drug treatment interruptions are prescribed by the doctor.

In addition, side effects should be carefully monitored, especially extrapyramidal symptoms and weight gain (see also paragraph, "Nutritional notes in TS").

In light of the described complications, a TS doctor should be reliable, available and expert. It is hard to find these three qualities in the same doctor, and as a consequence, some patients are not properly treated. The positive qualities of TS patients are at risk (e.g. creativity in Chapter 6), which could be socially enhanced with appropriate treatments.

Nutritional notes in TS

Considering TS and nutrition, two main aspects have to be discussed:

1 microbiota in TS
2 drug side effects and nutritional counselling

Microbiota in TS

Gut microbiota – microorganisms colonising the gut (see Chapter 2) – is affected by specific foods and dietary habits (Liu et al, 2015), which establish an interaction between diet, gut microbiota and the brain (Briguglio et al, 2018a). If adequately administered in the form of probiotic supplements, microbiota provides benefits to patients. Moreover, in some TS people, drugs, such as Risperidone, alter these microorganisms (Bahr et al, 2015). Dietary modifications or probiotic supplements are therefore employed in TS treatment. Nevertheless, TS microbiota need to be investigated through further robust studies.

Drug side effects and nutritional counselling

Nutritional counselling is required especially in TS low compliance patients (see below paragraph, "Compliance"). The goal is to inform patients about connections between the syndrome, the assumption of pharmacological treatments and the patient's nutritional status (Briguglio et al, 2018b). Depending on drug types, usual nutritional side effects in TS are:

- metabolic alterations.
- increased (or more rarely, decreased) appetite.
- body weight gain or changes in body structure.
- dry mouth and altered taste.
- constipation or other gastrointestinal disturbances.

TS case-by-case nutritional counselling (e.g. correct physical activity, meal timing, fibre intake) resolves these predictable side effects, preventing health risks (e.g. diabetes mellitus, cardiovascular diseases).

Table 4.11 Factors interfering with TS nutrition-related compliance (Porta, 1998; Briguglio et al, 2017).

☐ Fear of side effects of drugs
☐ Family environment affecting food habits
☐ Displeasure of body image
☐ Failure of previous diets

In childhood, poor food habits are common (Kuzbicka & Rachon, 2013). These habits risk turning into fattening and metabolic alterations, and they may also hide other pathologies. In these cases, patients have to be followed up by a nutritionist.

Eating habits (Box 4.1) are strongly connected with the family environment and the parental education. Readers should know that the prevalence of obesity among relatives of TS patients is four times higher than among controls (Comings & Comings, 1990).

Food habits are also affected through TS psychopathological mechanisms (e.g. OC component) and the consequent low compliance (Porta, 1998). In Table 4.11, the authors summarised all factors that alter nutrition-related compliance in TS patients. In these cases, the psychologist should collaborate with the nutritionist.

The implementation of teamwork (including also nutritional counselling and psychological support) is necessary for both patients and caregivers to enhance compliance, and provide accurate treatments.

Box 4.1   Nutritional habits in TS

TS patients and nutritional habits

Attitudes

An excessive speed of eating characterises TS patients, with the risk of being overweight, having a cardiometabolic alteration, or a liver disease (Briguglio et al, 2017). In severe cases, TS patients have binges (i.e. the ingestion of an abnormal quantity of food in a short period of time).

(continued)

(continued)

Timing

Some TS patients suffer from night eating. This habit could lead to hyperphagia (i.e. excessive drive to consume food), which is present in at least one third of TS sufferers. Obesity is a concrete danger for these patients.

Food preferences

A poor quality diet is often concomitant to unhealthy food choices in TS (Müller-Vahl et al, 2008). TS' heightened sensitivity to external stimuli (Belluscio et al, 2011) influences food preferences: taste is usually the first criterion of choice. Consequently, it has to be remarked that an excessive intake of sugars causes mood fluctuations and impulsivity. Alcohol abuse has a depressant effect, whereas caffeine abuse results in increased anxiety. A correct TS diet should balance the intake of carbohydrates, fats, proteins, fruits. For instance, impulsive eating will decrease by consuming healthy snacks (e.g. fresh fruits) in-between meals (Briguglio et al, 2017).

Nutritional supplements

These substances may contain vitamins, minerals and macro-molecules (e.g. carbohydrates) interacting with drug intake. Nutritional supplements' use is prevalent in American TS patients (Mantel et al, 2004). Professionals and caregivers should investigate any abusage that may compromise drugs' intake and compliance, with a special eye for sufferers with an altered body image perception.

Mini-invasive and surgical treatments

Botulinum toxin and Deep Brain Stimulation (DBS) are two possible, exceptional, treatment options for severe adult TS patients, being refractory to other medications and cognitive behavioural therapies, and suffering from a high Social Impairment burden (cf. Figure 4.8). These two treatments are mini-invasive procedures – namely, botulinum toxin – as they have a very low risk of harming the patient.

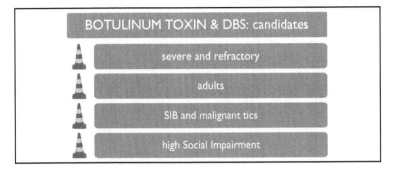

Figure 4.8 Candidates' criteria for botulinum toxin and DBS.
Credit: Cecilia Spalletti.

They have been offered to a few cases of severe TS minors in whom tics were causing self-injuries (cf. Figure 4.8).

Botulinum toxin

Botulinum toxin is a neurotoxin used with medical purposes. It is injected into the interested muscles to get a local release. In this way, the toxin blocks the tic process (see Chapter 2). Its effect lasts for about three to six months. Botulinum toxin needs, therefore, only a few injections a year (fewer than both Habit Reversal Training and the pharmacological treatment).

The downside of the toxin is that it can be used only for some specific simple and stable tics. It is employed especially in vocal tics, tongue tics and eye tics.

It may be used in adolescents and adults, whereas it is not well accepted by children because of their typical aversion to injections. Additionally, children's tics often change the body area, and therefore, they might be not suitable for botulinum toxin. This treatment may anyway be recommended in few minors suffering from malignant tics and SIB (Figure 4.8).

Deep Brain Stimulation

It has to be stressed that this intervention is used in adult patients. DBS is a mini-invasive and reversible neurosurgical procedure consisting in implanting two electrodes to stimulate specific brain nuclei of the patient (Porta et al, 2016; Figure 4.9). It is an experimental procedure, which resets pathological circuits related to tics and OC component (Visser-Vandewalle et al, 1999). Given the results – YGTSS score (see Chapter 3) decreases of 34% on average after DBS (Servello et al, 2016a; Servello et al, 2016b) – European Guidelines for Tourette syndrome approve DBS intervention for rare, severe and refractory adult TS patients (Müller-Vahl et al, 2011). Ad-hoc inclusions and exclusion criteria limit the eligibility of TS patients for this treatment (Porta et al, 2013).

Alert!

Children are not suitable for Deep Brain Stimulation!

Deep Brain Stimulation in TS plays an important role in controlling symptoms and in improving QoL. Moreover, DBS surgery has helped the scientific community in the understanding of the TS functioning (cf. Chapter 2; Priori et al, 2013).

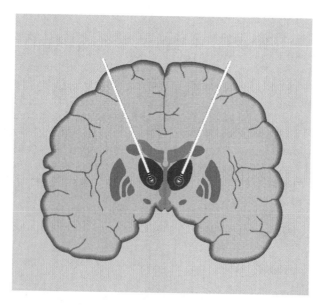

Figure 4.9 DBS in TS: a rare treatment for adult, severe and refractory patients.

Credit: Cecilia Spalletti.

Because of the variability of TS symptoms (cf. Chapter 3), the electrical neurostimulation is tailored to the specific patient's needs. In patients with predominant tics, the thalamus is recommended as target, whereas limbic targets are preferred in TS patients with predominant OC component (Porta et al, 2016).

Following the surgical procedure, the patient is guided by TS experts, who adapt psychological/ pharmacological treatments, and DBS setting, while monitoring symptoms' improvement. Regarding psychological treatments, a support is offered to patients and caregivers before and after surgery.

Other treatments

Innovative treatments are being studied for TS spectrum.

Considering psychological interventions, *bio(neuro) feedback* is a possible treatment for the future. Its aim is to self-direct and modulate specific areas of brain electrical activity, thanks to positive rewards, i.e. feedback, to the patient in case of success.

Group sessions, self-help groups, and Internet-based sessions are active treatments, but still under research.

Other treatments in TS are:

- in cases of TS related to streptococcal or viral infection: *plasmapheresis and intravenous immunoglobulin* (medical procedure, which consists in the exchange of blood plasma), *prednisolone* (steroid), *acyclovir* (antiviral agent), *ceftriaxone* (antibiotic).
- *clomifene, flutamide and finasteride* (hormonal therapies).
- new pharmacological agents in clinical research such as *deutetrabenazine* (monoamine depletor), which has been studied in the last two years with promising efficacy.
- *transcranial magnetic stimulation*, i.e. electromagnetic induction causing an electric current flux in a target brain region of the TS patient.
- *laser therapy*, i.e. infrared laser blood irradiation treating the antioxidative system of TS.

Alert!

No drug adjustments may be made without a TS doctor's approval.

The aforementioned treatments encounter an obstacle: the typical low compliance (Porta, 1998; Porta & Sironi, 2016) of TS patients.

Compliance

The word "compliance" means the patient and caregivers' adherence to clinicians' prescriptions during the diagnostic-therapeutic process.
Prescriptions mainly include:

- exams and visits to develop the diagnosis.
- dosage/time of drug taking and other drugs' proper instructions
- follow-up visit schedules.
- homework instructions when the patient is doing psychotherapy.
- hospital rules during recovery.

For example, prescriptions are not followed if a patient changes drug dosage without consulting the specialist. Another example is the lack of respect for the time of day to take the drug.
Compliance is divided into:

- Active or passive.

  1 Active: when the patient is deciding for his own healthcare, as generally happens for adults (for example, if an adult consciously decides not to take his own drug, it is a personal responsibility, therefore compliance is actively low).
  2 Passive: when the patient is not deciding for his own healthcare, as generally happens for children (for example, a parent doesn't give drugs to his child, therefore the patient's compliance is passively low). In case of severe pathologies, compliance is also passively low (for example, a severe depressed patient doesn't take his pills because of apathy). Another case of passive low compliance is when patients are forced to follow a therapy by someone else for example, by a judge or a family doctor.

- High, medium or low compliance: in relation with the level of accuracy when respecting prescriptions. Medium and low compliance lead to poor or no treatment effects, or even, in some cases, to the appearance of side effects.

N.B. TS patients' compliance is often medium to low. Let's find out the reason behind it. Impulsivity/compulsions and depressive symptoms play a negative role in the respect of rules, even when linked with one's own healthcare. Impulsivity/compulsions can lead to an altered drug dosage. Depression symptoms can include apathy and pessimism, and a patient can therefore decide to interrupt – temporary or indefinitely – a treatment.

Even perfectionism and pathological doubt are against compliance. It is hard for a patient with these symptoms to put his trust in someone else, caregivers and doctors included. Specifically, drug side effects and/or the fear of experiencing side effects are the primary cause of drug discontinuations (Silva et al, 1996). TS families are often against psychotropic drugs, especially for children, because of their possible cognitive and psychological side effects.

When expectations are too high or too low towards the efficacy of a treatment, they also play a role in the patient's and caregiver's attitude (e.g. a mother having expectations that are too high towards a drug treatment might think his son will immediately recover. Without consulting the doctor, she could dangerously interrupt the medical treatment as she doesn't see a tic decrease after few days).

In order to improve TS compliance, clinicians should:

- inform the patient about the treatments' function and mechanism of action and possible side effects.
- involve caregivers in the diagnostic-therapeutic process as they can practically and psychologically support the patient.
- (if necessary) work on the compliance itself in psychotherapy.

Clinicians need to be contactable by phone as much as possible in order to raise TS patients' compliance. On the other hand, patients should respect doctors and call them only in case of emergency.

Alert!

Help your doctor and yourself by being a compliant patient!

Conclusions

TS therapy is as complex as the syndrome itself, even for experts. Each symptom requires a tailor-made and timely treatment. The overall goal is the improvement of Quality of Life and this can only be achieved by teamwork; low compliance often represents an obstacle for a proper therapy. Treatments are also hard to be followed because of few centres dedicated to this "orphan" syndrome, high costs and off-label drugs.

A better knowledge of TS diagnostic-therapeutic pathways is needed between medical and social contexts to offer new options to these patients, their families and all the stakeholders.

References

Azrin NH & Nunn RG. 1973. Habit-reversal: A method of eliminating nervous habits and tics. Vol 11(4). *Behavioral Research and Therapy*, 619–628.

Azrin NH & Peterson AL. 1988. Habit reversal for the treatment of Tourette Syndrome. Vol 26(4). *Behavioral Research and Therapy*, 347–351.

Bahr SM., Tyler BC, Wooldridge N, Butcher BD, Burns TL, Teesch LM . . . , & Calarge CA. 2015. Use of the second-generation antipsychotic, risperidone, and secondary weight gain are associated with an altered gut microbiota in children. Vol 5. *Translational Psychiatry*, e652.

Belluscio BA, Jin L, Watters V, Lee TH, & Hallett M. 2011. Sensory sensitivity to external stimuli in Tourette syndrome patients. Vol 26(14). *Movement Disorders*, 2538–2543.

Bernstein DA & Borkovec TD. 1973. *Progressive Relaxation Training*. Champaign, IL, USA: Research Press, 11–50.

Borison RL, Ang L, Hamilton WJ, Diamond BI, & Davis JM. Treatment approaches in Gilles de la Tourette syndrome. 1983. Vol 11(2). *Brain Research Bulletin*, 205–208.

Briguglio M, Dell'Osso B, Galentino R, Zanaboni Dina C, Banfi G, & Porta M. 2017. Tics and obsessive-compulsive disorder in relation to diet: Two case reports. Vol 44(5). *Encephale*, 479–481.

Briguglio M, Dell'Osso B, Panzica G, Malgaroli A, Banfi G, Zanaboni Dina C, . . . , & Porta M. 2018a. Dietary neurotransmitters: A narrative review on current knowledge. Vol 10(5) *Nutrients*. pii: E591.

Briguglio M, Hrelia S, Malaguti M, Serpe L, Canaparo R, Dell'Osso B, . . . , & Banfi G. 2018b. Food bioactive compounds and their interference in drug pharmacokinetic/pharmacodynamic profiles. Vol 10(4). *Pharmaceutics*. pii: E277. Review.

Bruun RD & Budman CL. 1996. Risperidone as a treatment for Tourette's syndrome. Vol 57(1). *Journal of Clinical Psychiatry*, 29–31.

Cannon WB. 1929. *Bodily Changes in Pain, Hunger, Fear, and Rage*. Moscow, Russia: Ripol Classic Publishing House, 188–293.

Cath DC, Hedderly T, Ludolph AG, Stern JS, Murphy T, Hartmann A, . . . , & ESSTS Guidelines Group. 2011. European clinical guidelines for Tourette syndrome and other tic disorders. Part I: Assessment. Vol 20(4). *European Child and Adolescent Psychiatry*, 155–171.

Cavanna AE, Eddy CM, Mitchell R, Pall H, Mitchell I, Zrinzo L, . . . , & Rickards H. 2011. An approach to deep brain stimulation for severe treatment-refractory Tourette syndrome: The UK perspective. Vol 25(1). *British Journal of Neurosurgery*, 38–44.

Chappell PB, Leckman JF, & Riddle MA. 1995. The Pharmacological Treatment of Tic Disorders. Vol 4. *Child and Adolescent Psychiatric Clinic of North America*, 197–216.

Clark DM & Wells A. 1995. A cognitive model of social phobia. In: Heimberg R, Liebowitz M, Hope DA, & Schneier FR. *Social Phobia: Diagnosis, Assessment and Treatment*. New York, NY, USA: Guilford Press, 69–93.

Cohen DJ, Detlor J, Young JG, & Shaywitz BA. 1980. Clonidine ameliorates Gilles de la Tourette syndrome. Vol 37(12). *Archives of General Psychiatry*, 1350–1357.

Comings DE & Comings BG. 1990. A controlled family history study of Tourette's syndrome, II: Alcoholism, drug abuse, and obesity. Vol 51(7). *Journal of Clinical Psychiatry*, 281–287.

Dutta N & Cavanna AE. 2013. The effectiveness of habit reversal therapy in the treatment of Tourette syndrome and other chronic tic disorders: A systematic review. Vol 28(1). *Functional Neurology*, 7–12.

Eddy CM, Rickards HE, & Cavanna AE. 2011. Treatment strategies for tics in Tourette syndrome. Vol 4(1). *Therapeutic Advances in Neurological Disorders*, 25–45.

Goodman WK, Foote KD, Greenberg BD, Ricciuti N, Bauer R, Ward H, . . . , & Okun MS. 2010. Deep brain stimulation for intractable obsessive compulsive disorder: Pilot study using a blinded, staggered-onset design. Vol 67(6). *Biological Psychiatry*, 535–542.

Hanley GP, Iwata B, & McCord B. 2003. Functional analysis of problem behavior: a review. Vol 36(2). *Journal of Applied Behavioral Analysis*, 147–185.

Holmberg N & Kähkönen S. 2011. Internet-based cognitive-behavioural therapy in the treatment of psychiatric disorders. Vol 127. *Duodecim*, 692–698.

Jacobson E. 1938. *Progressive Relaxation*. Chicago, IL, USA: University of Chicago Press, 19–22 and 404.

Jankovic J & Kurlan R. 2011. Tourette syndrome: Evolving concepts. Vol 26(6). *Movement Disorders*, 1149–56.

Kuzbicka K & Rachon D. 2013. Bad eating habits as the main cause of obesity among children. Vol 19(3). *Pediatric Endocrinology*, 106–110.

Liu X, Cao S, & Zhang X. 2015. Modulation of gut microbiota-brain axis by probiotics, prebiotics, and diet. Vol 63(26). *Journal of Agricultural and Food Chemistry*, 7885–7895.

Lum LC. 1977. Breathing exercises in the treatment of hyperventilation and chronic anxiety states. Vol 2. *Chest, Heart and Stroke Journal*, 6–11.

Mantel BJ, Meyers A, Tran QY, Rogers S, & Jacobson JS. 2004. Nutritional supplements and complementary/alternative medicine in Tourette syndrome. Vol 14(4). *Journal of Child and Adolescent Psychopharmacology*, 582–589.

McGuire JF, Ricketts EJ, Piacentini J, Murphy TK, Storch EA, & Lewin AB. 2015. Behavior therapy for Tic disorders: An evidenced-based review and new directions for treatment research. Vol 2. *Current Developmental Disorders Reports*. 309–317.

Müller-Vahl KR, Buddensiek N, Geomelas M, & Emrich HM. 2008. The influence of different food and drink on tics in Tourette syndrome. Vol 97(4). *Acta Paediatrica*, 442–446.

Müller-Vahl KR, Cath DC, Cavanna AE, Dehning S, Porta M, Robertson MM, . . . , & ESSTS Guidelines Group. 2011. European clinical guidelines for Tourette syndrome and other tic disorders. Part IV: Deep brain stimulation. Vol 20(4). *European Child & Adolescent Psychiatry*, 209–217.

Peterson AL & Azrin NH. 1992. An evaluation of behavioral treatments for Tourette syndrome. Vol 30(2). *Behavior Research and Therapy*, 167–174.

Piacentini J, Woods DW, Scahill L, Wilhelm S, Peterson AL, Chang S, . . . , & Walkup JT. 2010. Behavior therapy for children with Tourette disorder: a randomized controlled trial. Vol 303(19). *JAMA*, 1929–1937.

Porta M. 1998. *La compliance in neurologia*. Torino, IT, EU: Utet Periodici Scientifici.

Porta M, Cavanna AE, Zekaj E, D'Adda F, & Servello D. 2013. Selection of patients with Tourette syndrome for deep brain stimulation surgery. Vol 27(1). *Behavioral Neurology*, 125–131.

Porta M, Saleh C, Zekaj E, Zanaboni Dina C, Bona AR, Servello D. 2016. Why so many deep brain stimulation targets in Tourette's syndrome? Toward a broadening of the definition of the syndrome. Vol 123(7). *Journal of Neural Transmission*, 785–790.

Porta M & Sironi VA. 2016. *Il Cervello Irriverente: La sindrome di Tourette, la malattia dei mille tic*. Bari, IT, EU: Laterza Editori, 161.

Priori A, Giannicola G, Rosa M, Marceglia S, Servello D, Sassi M, & Porta M. 2013. Deep brain electrophysiological recordings provide clues to the pathophysiology of Tourette syndrome. Vol 37(6). *Neuroscience and Biobehavioral Reviews*, 1063–1068.

Pringsheim T, Doja A, Gorman D, McKinlay D, Day L, Billinghurst L, . . . , & Sandor P. 2012. Canadian guidelines for the evidence-based treatment of tic disorders: Pharmacotherapy. Vol 57(3). *Canadian Journal of Psychiatry*, 133–143.

Robertson MM. 2000. Tourette Syndrome, associated conditions and the complexities of treatment. Vol 123. *Brain*, 425–462.

Roessner V, Rothenberger A, Rickards H, & Hoekstra PJ. 2011a. European clinical guidelines for Tourette syndrome and other tic disorders. Vol 20(4). *European Child & Adolescent Psychiatry*,153–154.

Roessner V, Plessen KJ, Rothenberger A, Ludolph AG, Rizzo R, Skov L, . . . , & ESSTS Guidelines Group. 2011b. European clinical guidelines for Tourette syndrome and other tic disorders. Part II: pharmacological treatment. Vol 20(4) *European Child & Adolescent Psychiatry*, 173–196.

Sallee FR, Nesbitt L, Jackson C, Sine L, & Sethuraman G. 1997. Relative efficacy of Haloperidol and Pimozide in children and adolescents with Tourette's disorder. Vol 154(8) *American Journal of Psychiatry*, 1057–1062.

Sandor P, Musisi S, Moldofsky H, & Lang A. 1990. Tourette syndrome: A follow-up study. Vol 10(3). *Journal of Clinical Psychopharmacology*, 197–199.

Sandor P & Carroll A. 2012. Canadian guidelines for the evidence-based treatment of tic disorders. Vol 57(3). *Canadian Journal of Psychiatry*, 131–132.

Scalone L, D'Angiolella LS, Mantovani LG, Galentino R, Servello D, Dell'Osso B, . . . , & Porta M. 2017. Obsessive Compulsive Tic Disorder: Appropriate diagnosis and treatment as key elements to improve health and rationalize use of resources. Vol 14(4). *Epidemiology Biostatistics and Public Health*, e12661-9.

Servello D, Zekaj E, Saleh C, Zanaboni Dina C, & Porta M. 2016a. Sixteen years of deep brain stimulation in Tourette's Syndrome: A critical review. Vol 60(2). *Journal of Neurosurgical Sciences*, 218–229.

Servello D, Zekaj E, Saleh C, Lange N, & Porta M. 2016b. Deep Brain Stimulation in Gilles de la Tourette Syndrome: What Does the Future Hold? A Cohort of 48 Patients. Vol 78(1). *Neurosurgery*, 91–100.

Silva RR, Munoz DM, Daniel W, Barickman J, & Friedhoff AJ. 1996. Causes of haloperidol discontinuation in patients with Tourette's disorder: Management and alternatives. Vol 57(3). *Journal of Clinical Psychiatry*, 129–135.

Singer HS. 2010. Treatment of tics and Tourette syndrome. Vol 12(6). *Current Treatment Options in Neurology*, 539–561.

Steeves T, McKinlay BD, Gorman D, Billinghurst L, Day L, Carroll A, Dion Y, Doja A, Luscombe S, Sandor P, & Pringsheim T. 2012. Canadian guidelines for the evidence-based treatment of tic disorders: Behavioural therapy, deep brain stimulation, and transcranial magnetic stimulation. Vol 57(3). *Canadian Journal of Psychiatry*, 144–151.

Verdellen C, van de Griendt J, Hartmann A, Murphy T, & ESSTS Guidelines Group. 2011. European clinical guidelines for Tourette syndrome and other tic disorders. Part III: Behavioural and psychosocial interventions. Vol 20(4). *European Child and Adolescent Psychiatry*, 197–207.

Vandewalle V, van der Linden C, Groenewegen HJ, & Caemaert J. 1999. Stereotactic treatment of Gilles de la Tourette syndrome by high frequency stimulation of thalamus. Vol 353(9154). *Lancet*, 724.

Woods DW, Piacentini J, Chang S, Deckersbach T, Ginsburg GS, Peterson AL, . . . , & Wilhelm S. 2008. *Managing Tourette Syndrome. A behavioural intervention for children and adults. Therapist Guide*. New York, NY, USA: Oxford University Press, 19–114.

Chapter 5

The role of family*

Summary

Family plays a key role in the management of Tourette syndrome patients, from the communication of the diagnosis through to the treatments. Parental compliance should therefore be high as it will have a positive influence on the patient. Family is "the place" where symptoms increase; parents, siblings and partners may be involved, thus affecting relationships. When other members have TS symptoms as well, family functioning is more complicated.

TS team has the task to inform family members about TS features, providing them with behavioural recommendations. Parent Training is the ad hoc intervention for those families who need to be followed when facing TS daily issues, including how to deal with the education of sufferers.

Introduction

"Family functioning" refers to the skills of family members to promote and sustain the overall well-being of the home environment. Being in a peaceful family context helps to develop functional emotional regulation more than other social contexts could, or the child by himself could (Bronfenbrenner, 1986). In family relationships, stressful stimuli ("barriers") are balanced by supporting each other (facilitating mechanisms) (Belsky, 1984). On the other hand, parental stress can affect the quality of relationships, giving origin to a Social Impairment of the child (Benzies et al, 2004). A child suffering from a medical condition can increase the level of parental stress, and as a consequence, this can exacerbate the child's state of illness.

* In collaboration with Roberta Galentino

Stressful stimuli associated with Tourette syndrome are those also found in other medical conditions, such as coping with the diagnosis or managing routine changes. Excessive parental responsibility, difficulty in carrying out domestic activities, and lack of communication between parents and TS children are also reported (Matthews et al, 1985).

TS family functioning is often poor, and it is associated with the psychosocial adaptation of the child (Robertson et al, 1988). Mothers of TS children in particular suffer low self-esteem, when compared with control mothers, and this consequently influences the TS child's self-esteem (Edell-Fisher & Motta, 1990; Carter et al, 2000).

As seen in the previous chapters, TS symptoms increase at home and psychopathologies, when compared with tics, are more likely to have an impact on family life. It is not rare that exhausted parents or partners, no longer able to bear TS symptoms (e.g. obsessions toward a family member), would request that the sufferer is referred to a Tourette Centre. This often happens even before the patient understands that he has a disorder.

In the next paragraphs, the most common concerns affecting the family are explained:

- Acceptance of diagnosis and compliance.
- Family reactions in front of tics.
- Educating TS children.
- Managing sibling relationships.
- TS couples' conflicts.

At least 50% of the aforementioned concerns are easily found in any family. The main difference between a family and a family with a TS person is that, at first, relatives are not aware about best behaviours to adopt to make the patient feel better. Before being followed by a TS team, relatives sometimes either underestimate or underline excessively the sufferer's symptoms, without sorting any positive effect, or even increasing the patient's diseases. After the diagnosis, treatment options (cf. Chapter 4) are explained to TS families and clinicians guide each member through behavioural recommendations. The final goals of involving families in TS treatments are:

1   promoting the sufferer's wellness
2   preventing from family conflicts
3   strengthen family connections

The acceptance of diagnosis and compliance

When the diagnosis is given, family members can have different types of reactions (Khoury, 2017). Children's naivety often makes the youngest member(s) more likely to accept the disease. On the other hand, the kind of family approach to the disease, and its related behaviours, influences children's reaction. Parents, especially mothers, are usually the most responsive; they often feel discomfort about thinking of the consequences on their child's life. They worry about their own ability to manage the situation at home, and they are preoccupied with the idea of their child being properly medically treated, and that he could become a victim of social discrimination (Malli et al, 2016).

Parents may show these different reactions in front of diagnosis (Haerle, 1992):

- Experiencing a sense of guilt, especially when the parent has himself tics (Leckman & Cohen, 1999). This may result in family dysfunctional changes, for example a mother of a TS sufferer abandoning all her hobbies as a consequence of her thinking the more she spends time with the child the better he will feel. Parental support has to be considered.
- On the contrary, thanks to the diagnosis, some parents are relived from their sense of guilt, and feel that they can finally give a name to their son's disturbances (Woods et al, 2007). Until that moment, they are unable to explain the reason of the sufferer's disease.
- In more difficult cases, the family reacts by denying the diagnosis (Robertson et al, 1988) because of the shock it causes (e.g. when the syndrome suddenly appears, or when family conditions are already complicated). With a neglectful attitude, parents could start looking for distractions, without following experts' suggestions (i.e. low compliance, cf. Chapter 4). Psychological intervention is mandatory, even because of the implications on the patient's acceptance and compliance.
- Sadness can precede and/or accompany parental acceptance (Rivera-Navarro et al, 2009). If a pathological mood persists, parents are invited to follow a psychological treatment.

From diagnosis onwards, family members and clinicians should collaborate with specific tasks:

- Experts should inform the family about the fundamental TS aspects: treatment options, drugs' side effects, agenda management, syndrome's evolution and spontaneous remission. Experts should equip the family with books, scientific papers, and put them in contact with TS associations and other sufferers.
- Family should share emotions, especially fears, with the other members, with friends or specialists, in order to feel supported, and to create an extended environment for the child: he will feel less anxious and more accepted when exhibiting tics and behavioural problems.

Alert!

Trust your TS team and follow recommendations! Your child will have an earlier recovery.

Compliance (cf. Chapter 4) benefits from these tasks, if they are respected and maintained for the whole diagnostic-therapeutic pathway. A high family compliance is more likely to generate a medium or high child's compliance. Compliance is fundamental for TS experts to balance their interventions and, therefore, for the patient to be early and properly treated.

Differences on diagnosis' acceptance are also based on the sociocultural features of the sufferer's family. In this book, other influencing contexts for the sufferer coping the diagnostic phase are presented, for example school (Chapter 6) and friends (Chapter 7).

Family reactions in front of tics

A correct response in front of tics is essential for a positive family life. Clinicians provide behavioural suggestions for families, and TS associations groups do so for parents in family meetings. They can benefit from mutual support while receiving indications by experts. Families learn the correct management of the annoyance caused by hearing or seeing frequent abnormal sounds or movements. It is essential for every member of the family to ignore tics. To underline the manifestation of tics or to comment on it, causes an increased level of stress that will, in turn, exacerbate tics (Haerle, 1992).

Moreover, a tic can worsen if its response is an unusual display of affection, a laugh, or even a smile. They are positive reinforcements for the child!

Alert!

Ignore your child's tics.

Even if the best option is to ignore tics, often it feels exhausting to do so. For this reason, experts should present it clearly as the best practice for families to follow, and congratulate those who already manage it.

Some tics can't be ignored, e.g. frequent spitting, and they need other ad hoc recommendations.

Before being informed, parents can develop feelings of guilt for not knowing how to deal with outbursts. This can sometimes lead to the use of aggressive tones and manners (Leckman & Cohen, 1999). To increase the tolerance threshold, parents can try to focus on something else or look for other strategies. As an example, a young sister of a TS patient could move to another room if she is having a hard time in ignoring the brother's tic arrival.

It is very important for each member of the family to have their own space at home (e.g. to read quietly), spare time and social life (Figure 5.2). This is helpful for the personal Quality of Life and for reducing stress related to the assistance given to the TS sufferer.

By monitoring tics during the day, families realise triggers and reactions, taking also into account their own role in reinforcing or reducing tics. Parents should also monitor the quality of their own responses when tics occur in public. By doing so, parents allow the child with TS to accept his condition and feel more "at ease". In case parents feel the urge to change their attitude, they should consult an expert (Woods et al, 2008).

Educating TS children

Data literature show how stressing is for parents to educate children with TS (Robinson et al, 2013). The inability to distinguish and manage between the TS behavioural issue and the intention of their child is a recurrent doubt haunting TS parents, who are uncertain whether to educate or not. Parents frequently adopt different educational methods, shifting too fast from one to another as soon as they do not see any improvements (Gurman & Kniskern, 1995). The tendency of justifying or being too compassionate is often practiced by parents in order to avoid further discussions or outbursts of rage (Barkley, 1997). This over protective attitude towards children may limit their ability to develop autonomy, resulting in an adult being less capable of taking responsibility for his actions.

Alert!

Education should be as thorough as for non-TS children.

Parents need to maintain their authority, even to promote a positive compliance to treatments.

Recommendations to better educate the TS child (Woods et al, 2007):

- Reinforce (with praises, smiles or prizes) the child's acting in the right way, without being too tough when their behaviour is not as expected. Rewarding is more motivating than sanctions!

    Of course, corporal punishment would only increase the aggressive attitudes of the child. He would be encouraged to think that the use of violence is a problem-solving option.

    N.B. The use of reinforcement after positive behaviours should be random, so as to avoid the child to think every positive behaviour will be rewarded. This would instead increase the TS patient's pursuit of perfectionism.
- Involve children in setting rules and deciding sanctions when rules are not followed.
- Set up a "structured" daily routine in order to avoid unexpected changes that usually generate stress (with a consequent tic increase). It would be advisable to follow routines even during holidays (see also Chapter 7).

It is suggested to be optimistic rather than "catastrophic" in order to resist the temptation of being over-protective. Families should carry out the same old activities, including spending time together, practicing sports and deal with house chores, in order to teach the child that he is still able to conduct a normal life, without duties being put aside.

Sibling relationships

Another aspect that complicates the family functioning is the relationship between the child suffering from TS and his brothers and sisters (Lebowitz & Scahill, 2013; Figure 5.1). TS patients' siblings may experience different parental treatments: they feel less considered, left alone in their daily activities, or expected to be more autonomous and responsible even when younger. After TS onset, increased conflicts between siblings are not infrequent. Jealousies and feelings of anger may rise, caused by lack of attention (Woods et al, 2007). For these reasons, parents should always find special moments for each child, thus distributing attentions and responsibilities equally. Sometimes the sibling feels too much responsibility for their TS brother or sister and develops an excessive sense of protection that could for example result in mood disturbances, characterised by anger or sadness. Moreover, a young teenager could be embarrassed about the sibling's tics, especially in social contexts (Woods et al, 2007).

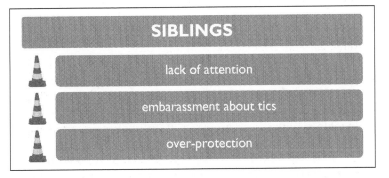

Figure 5.1 Main problems regarding siblings of TS children.
Credit: Cecilia Spalletti.

Feeling embarrassed by the sibling's tics, or being over-protective, could result in the progressive abandonment of activities. A child could avoid inviting his friends over or may not like to take part in family plans anymore.

It is essential after the diagnosis, to explain the medical condition and consequences to all members of the family, in particular to siblings. It is important to underline that tics are impossible to control, and not contagious. Siblings, as with mums and dads, should be explained that it is advised to ignore tics as much as possible. When ignoring tics may be difficult for siblings, it could be useful to provide moments and spaces to be separate from them, such as when studying or playing. It is only in rare and severe cases that OC component plays against sibling relationship, forcing them to be separated in two different homes. In the case of a TS child maltreating his siblings, it would be essential to immediately correct the behaviour with the help of a TS expert.

N.B: pets may be victim of OC component as well, and in severe cases they could need to leave the home.

Techniques from Parent Training

Studies show that enhanced long-lasting relationships between parents and TS children, reduce stress and improve their behavioural problems (Robinson et al, 2013). Treatment often includes behavioural interventions, in addition to drugs or not, resulting in positive outcomes for the whole family psychological wellbeing. Some treatments are addressed to mothers and fathers, i.e. Parent Training (see also Chapter 4). TS Parent Training should include:

- Information about TS nature and difficulties that may be encountered by parents.
- Development of positive parental approaches with a focus on the global life of the family, and not only on the disease of the child.

Knowledge and recommendations are helpful to manage TS conditions and to not become a victim of the syndrome (Hansen, 1992; Porta, 2013).

Alert!

Parents may have different approaches to the syndrome.

It is advisable for parents to cooperate as a team.

Parents are guided by the psychologist to practice, once home, some techniques aiming to improve specific behavioural aspects of their child within the family context (Foxx, 2014). The most used techniques are: diary and ABC, token economy, time out, ad hoc instructions, sharing of the rules.

Diary and ABC

As in Observation and in Habit Reversal Training (cf. Chapter 4), a monitoring system, namely a diary, is offered in Parent Training. This system allows parents to follow tics' and behavioural problems' frequency trend. A diary would be created and used by parents to record a specific symptom (chosen before as a target). It can be used together with ABC technique (cf. Chapter 4) with the aim of finding out antecedent causes (A), and to evaluate consequences (C), of the targeted symptom (B). If a greater frequency of the issue is detected as triggered by a specific cause, the parents, along with a psychologist, would investigate what happened, thus remodeling the situation to prevent from future severe bouts.

Token economy

When a child is improving their targeted behaviour, the parents are asked to reinforce them through a reward. Rewards may be family activities (e.g. a trip with grandparents, going to the park with mum), permissions (e.g. playing with favourite games, going to the cinema with friends) or presents (e.g. a new sticker album, a new t-shirt). The reward should be chosen by the child themselves in agreement with both parents. To use rewards more consistently, parents and children can create their own "token economy" (calling it with a funny name such as "Star System"). A daily, weekly or monthly list of positive actions has to be generated and a reward has to be chosen for motivating the child to reach the pre-set score. Each positive behaviour could be worth 1 point or more and the prize could be awarded only when the score is reached. It is important that the compensation (points) is given immediately after the action, otherwise the child may not be able to link the prize with the behaviour itself. N.B. Token economy has a different reinforce model from educational system (cf. paragraph, "Educating TS children").

A billboard can be used to keep track of the positive behaviours carried out and to mark with points (Table 5.1). A bonus could also be given for activities that are highly relevant for the family context. E.g. A severe ADHD child could be rewarded with a bonus for staying seated at the table with the whole family until the end of dinner.

Siblings often become jealous of attentions and prizes given to the TS sufferer through this technique. Parents should explain them the token economy's rationale, and pay attention to balance their care between offspring.

Another context where using the token economy technique is school (cf. Chapter 6).

Here are a few suggestions for the rewarding system:

• At the very beginning, in order to motivate the child, prizes can be reached within few days (e.g. five days). Once the first prize is assigned, the family can add more and more days to the next rewarding systems.
• Tasks, point systems and rewards should be very clear.

Table 5.1 Example of token economy. Robert was able to collect the preset 7 points in trying to do one thing at a time; the prize will be playing a baseball match with his dad on Sunday.

Robert's task: to do one thing at the time	————— lack of success	🌸 partial success	🌸🌸 success
Monday			🌸🌸
Tuesday			🌸🌸
Wednesday			🌸🌸
Thursday		🌸	
Friday	-------------------		
Goal: minimum 7/10 🌸	Reward: baseball match with dad on Sunday.		

- It is better to choose "affective" rewards (e.g. going to the cinema with mum, playing with a friend) rather than the "material" ones (e.g. buying a new game). In case of material prizes, it is likely that positive behaviours occur just because of the "barter".
- Once the reward system has become of use, parents can add "costs" in the event of a child not acting according to agreements. A child could be losing scores and rewards.
- This technique can also be used for modeling teenagers' behaviours, by adapting challenges and rewards.
- When the sufferer is mature enough to understand the advantage of appropriate behaviours, the system could become a pact between him and his parents, entailing fewer and fewer rewards.

Time out

This technique is generally indicated to stop children's dysfunctional behaviours (e.g. aggressive behaviours). When manifesting a negative conduct, the child has to spend a period of time alone in "time out" (e.g. 1 minute for each year of age) in a place without any pleasant incentive. After the "time out", parents could approach the child, making sure he understood the reason of the "time out", before allowing him to go back to his activities.

Ad hoc instructions

Parents can improve their management of child's negative behaviours by following ad hoc instructions:

- Reducing the rules to the minimum necessary.
- Using specific and clear rules.
- Being consistent (to show consequences as previously agreed with the child).

Sharing of the rules

When the age and the maturity of the child allow it, it is advised to include them in setting rules. They will feel like a co-builder of their own wellness, without impositions (often in contrast with behavioural problems such as oppositional defiant disorder). It is therefore useful to spend the necessary time with the child before approaching the targeted activity (e.g. when hosting guests), clearly reminding them about rules and consequences previously established.

Despite all difficulties, in mild cases Parent Training is not necessary: TS aspects can be managed by the child himself, with the help of a positive attitude, reinforcement and empowerment coming from family members.

The couple

Talking about the life as a couple, two different situations may be considered:

1   A couple having a child with TS.
2   A TS partner in a couple.

In the first case, TS issues can be a strain on the couple (Benzies et al, 2004). Partners should maintain their own space (Haerle, 1992) without neglecting any personal life sphere (see Figure 5.2,

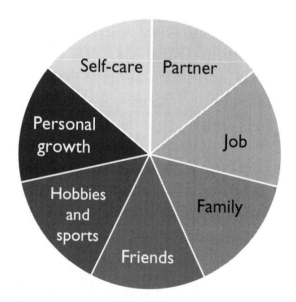

Figure 5.2 Adapted from Strocchi & Jodice (2000): personal life spheres.
Credit: Cecilia Spalletti.

cf. also Chapter 7). The devotion to the companion comes first, followed by friends, self-care, personal growth, having a job, hobbies and sport. All of those spheres help preserve the global well-being of a couple.

In case of adult patients, the couple can face the following issues:

1 The partner is bothered by tics (e.g. John's wife can't concentrate on her online course because John has a screaming tic).
2 The partner is involved in rituals (e.g. because of his OC component, Michael would spend an hour to set the table for two people, consequently his partner Samantha would start to do it on her own).
3 The partner complains about side effects of drugs (for example low sexual libido or lack of enthusiasm in doing something).

It is helpful for the partner to take part to the TS patient's visits. Clinicians can interview the companion to collect his considerations and improve the couple's Quality of Life.

Conclusions

Family is "where" the patient is born; often tics are also "born" in family because of relatives having their own TS symptoms. Family relationships cannot, in any instance, cause TS. High stress levels in families may increase existing symptoms.

TS families are guided by experts in promoting a higher Quality of Life of the patient through behavioural recommendations. Compliance is therefore essential to be respected by each member of the family as, one by one, they can give a contribute in the guise of parent, or sibling, or partner. Besides educating children, parents have the fundamental role of making an effort in accepting the syndrome. As a result, the entire family will adopt a unique positive attitude with regard to the disease.

References

Barkley RA. 1997. *Defiant Children. Second Edition. A Clinician's Manual for Assessment and Parent Training.* New York, NY, USA: The Guilford Press, 40–41.

Belsky J. 1984. The Determinants of Parenting: A Process Model. Vol 55(1). *Child Development*, 83–96.

Benzies KM, Harrison MJ, & Magill-Evans J. 2004. Parenting Stress, Marital Quality, and Child Behavior Problems at Age 7 Years. Vol 21(2). *Public Health Nursing*, 111–121.

Bronfenbrenner U. 1986. Ecology of the family as a context for human-development-research perspectives. Vol 22(6). *Developmental Psychology*, 723–742.

Carter AS, O'Donnell DA, Schultz RT, Scahill L, Leckman JF, & Pauls DL. 2000. Social and emotional adjustment in children affected with Gilles de la Tourette's syndrome: Associations with ADHD and family functioning. Attention Deficit Hyperactivity Disorder. Vol 41(2). *Journal of Child Psychology and Psychiatry*, 215–223.

Edell-Fisher BH & Motta RW. 1990. Tourette syndrome: Relation to children's and parents' self-concepts. Vol 66(2). *Psychological Reports*, 539–545.

Foxx RM. 2014. *Tecniche base del metodo comportamentale. Per l'handicap grave e l'autismo*. Trento, IT, EU: Erickson, 121–168.

Gurman AS & Kniskern DP. 1995. *Manuale di terapia della famiglia*. Torino, IT, EU: Bollati Boringhieri, 293–303.

Haerle T. 1992. Adjusting to your child's diagnosis. In: Hearle T, eds. *Children with Tourette Syndrome: A Parent's Guide*. Rockville, MD, USA: Woodbine House, 27–52.

Hansen CR. 1992. Children with Tourette syndrome and their families. In: Hearle T, eds. *Children with Tourette Syndrome: A Parents' Guide*. Rockville, MD, USA: Woodbine House, 113–138.

Khoury R. 2017. Mothers of children with Tourette's syndrome. Vol 19. *Interdisciplinary Contexts of Special Pedagogy*, 171–199.

Leckman JF & Cohen DJ. 1999. *Tourette's syndrome – Tics, Obsessions, Compulsions: Developmental Psychopathology and Clinical Care*. New York, NY, USA: John Wiley and Sons, 113, 357.

Malli MA, Forrester-Jones R, & Murphy G. 2016. Stigma in youth with Tourette's syndrome: A systematic review and synthesis. Vol 25(2). *European Child & Adolescent Psychiatry*, 127–139.

Lebowitz ER & Scahill L. 2013. Psychoeducational Interventions: What Every Parent and Family Member Need to Know. In: Martino D & Leckman JF, eds. *Tourette Syndrome*. Oxford, UK, EU: Oxford University Press, 496–497.

Matthews M, Eustace C, Grad G, Pelcovitz D, & Olson M. 1985. A family systems perspective on Tourette's Syndrome. Vol 6(1). *International Journal of Family Psychiatry*, 53–66.

Porta M. 2013. *Tic, Tourette e disturbi correlati. Manuale pratico d'uso*. Roma, IT, EU: CIC Edizioni Internazionali, 45–48.

Rivera-Navarro J, Cubo E, & Almazán J. 2009. The diagnosis of Tourette's Syndrome: Communication and impact. Vol 14(1). *Clinical Child Psychology and Psychiatry*, 13–23.

Robertson MM, Trimble MR, & Lees AJ. 1988. The Psychopathology of the Gilles De La Tourette Syndrome. Vol 152. *British Journal of Psychiatry*, 383–390.

Robinson LR, Bitsko RH, Schieve LA, & Visser SN. 2013. Tourette syndrome, parenting aggravation, and the contribution of co-occurring conditions among a nationally representative sample. Vol 6(1). *Disability Health Journal*, 26–35.

Strocchi MC & Jodice L. 2000. *La coppia che non scoppia. Educazione sentimentale*. Verona, IT, EU: Positive Press, 1–172.

Woods DW, Piacentini J, Chang S, Deckersbach T, Ginsburg G, Peterson A, . . . , Wilhelm S. 2008. *Managing Tourette Syndrome: A Behavioral Intervention. Parent Workbook. (Treatments That Work)*. Oxford, UK, EU: Oxford University Press, 9–36.

Woods DW, Piacentini J, Walkup JT. 2007. *Treating Tourette Syndrome and Tic Disorders: A Guide for Practitioners*. New York, NY, USA: The Guilford Press, 226, 228–231.

Chapter 6

The role of school*

Summary

School is the place where TS patients have the most control of symptoms. Social motivation (especially the relationship with schoolmates) is indeed a strong support to reduce tics, compulsions or other manifestations.

In many cases, clinicians equip teachers (and schoolmates) with guidance about homework, exams and other strategies to improve the biopsychosocial health of the TS student.

The prospect of a TS sufferer's working life is also described in this chapter, considering that patients, and their parents, are often afraid of having fewer opportunities. TS people must have as many possibilities as everyone else, and the law should support them.

Moreover, several TS patients have a higher level of creativity if compared with the general population. This skill can be a useful addition at school and at work.

Introduction

TS syndrome's prevalence is up to 18% among school children (see Chapter 3). The first tics usually appear between kindergarten and the primary school years, reaching their peak during secondary school. Then tics improve, and TS' behavioural characteristics stabilise in adulthood, when a person begins their working life (see paragraph, "After school life: working life").

During primary school, TS patients develop their first control skills and they become able to delay or suppress tics for a short

* In collaboration with Selenia Greco

period of time. Environmental or emotional conditions, such as school-related anxiety, may influence the tic manifestation (Conelea & Woods, 2008). For this reason, a positive school environment plays a key role in preventing the TS student's academic difficulties and, on a bigger scale, in promoting the TS student's psychosocial wellness (Wadman et al, 2016).

Before introducing any school-related information and suggestions to be used by teachers, it is important to remind families that a correct diagnosis is essential (cf. Chapter 3). It often happens that TS patients are wrongly diagnosed and treated as having ADHD or other diseases. Usually, at school, a mistaken diagnosis can lead to additional problems, such as:

- manifestation of untreated tics or OC component.
- manifestation of untreated depression or anxiety symptoms.
- high Social Impairment.
- low grades.
- following a personalised class curriculum based on the mistaken diagnosis.
- being moved to a different class/school even when not necessary.

Even if the TS behavioural symptoms are usually more impairing than tics, the connotation of the syndrome as Tic Disorder wrongly leads to putting these other symptoms aside. They don't get the attention they deserve, with negative consequences on school performance and on the social life of the student.

School is a "special" place for a child with TS. When at school, a child will consciously or unconsciously (see Figure 6.1) have more control on tics than when they are at home. On the other hand, this will lead to a greater consumption of energy. In addition to this huge effort, tic control will be reinforced or damaged by the quality of schoolmates' relationships and, moreover by the student's self-efficacy and self-esteem.

A TS student has to face various difficulties, not only those related to the fulfilment of school commitments. In addition to this, in severe patients, during the syndrome's peak periods or in some stressful moments of the day, control is not practicable. Even though a child's effort is the greatest, when they haven't got control of symptoms, they feel trapped in their own body, and feel inadequate and different from schoolmates.As a result, they will experience a sense of defect in self-esteem and self-efficacy (Silvestri et al, 2018; Figure 6.1).

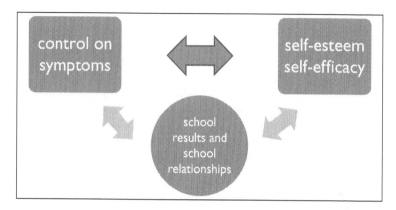

Figure 6.1 The majority of TS students are able to control symptoms in class with an effect on either school results and relationships. Self-esteem and self-efficacy play a role, as well.

Credit: Cecilia Spalletti.

A TS student has to face these challenges:

- controlling tics to avoid being mocked.
- dealing with inappropriate behaviours.
- working hard to remain at a good academic level and to stay on track with the class.

The good news is that this doesn't prevent TS students from performing successfully academically. It may only be a bit more difficult than for people not suffering from TS. Even if TS students have to spend more energy to obtain a similar result, their behaviours are often misinterpreted by schoolmates, who accuse them of being rude or lazy. On the other hand, when a teacher can't make positive changes, she may feel a sense of "learned helplessness" (Seligman, 1972). To prevent this, teachers, schoolmates and the sufferer themselves need to be supported by TS experts (Figure 6.2). This is the unique way in which school could become a peaceful place, enriching the child with positive experiences and be meaningful for all the school stakeholders. As a good consequence, the whole class will develop a better understanding of diversity and inclusion.

Having a sociocultural change to support TS people as a main goal, it is necessary to work on school intrapersonal and interpersonal processes. The main actors of these processes are:

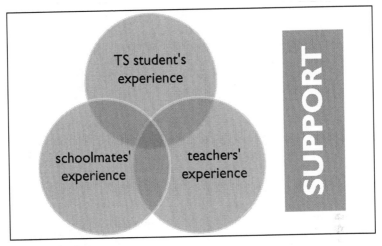

Figure 6.2 At school, support is needed for everyone as their experiences cross.
Credit: Cecilia Spalletti.

- the TS student
- schoolmates
- teachers

The following paragraphs are focused on the three school actors listed here.

Patient's experience

TS students can face a series of difficulties at school, both on the academic and social level. For this reason, many of these students could benefit from a special needs teacher and from ad hoc educational suggestions (see Table 6.6 at the end of the chapter). Even though, the IQ of a child with TS is on or above average, his scholastic experience is strongly influenced by therapies and by the support he receives. When TS is accompanied by behavioural diseases, a student is even more prone to have both academic difficulties and poor class relationships (Kadesjö & Gillberg, 2000): this more often requires a support.

In fact, tics are just one of the big obstacles for the sufferer at school; TS children often complain about:

- handwriting and eye tics.
- embarassment when performing sound tics, especially coprolalia.
- learning disorders mainly caused by attention deficit (attention is often shifted on tics/obsessions) and by hyperactivity (e.g. they hardly stay seated at the desk).
- performance anxiety, especially when reading out loud in front of the whole class.

Table 6.1 explains TS issues (with strong influence on educational life), divided by categories. N.B.: the order of Table 6.1 follows the frequency of the issues, from highly to less frequent.

Tics. Motor and sound tics mainly interfere with reading and writing. One of the most impairing tics at school is without doubt the handwriting tic. Also eye tics (blinking, staring into a specific direction; neck or shoulders' tics preventing from gazing) will make it difficult to read and write without interruptions. Many strategies may be adopted to support the TS student for both handwriting and eye tics (see Table 6.6).

Other types of tics have more influence on TS students' relationships (Sukhodolsky et al, 2003). The more the tic is visible or audible by others, the more the relationship may be "disturbed" by tics. Sound tics are generally more annoying than motor tics for the student's schoolmates. Moreover, copropraxia and coprolalia (i.e. coprophenomena)

Table 6.1 TS issues with strong influence on school life.

Category	Issue
Tics	motor tics
	sound tics
Neurobehavioural diseases	ADHD
	OC component
	learning disorders
Psychological diseases	anxiety
	school phobia
	depression
Other issues	homework
	NOSI and oppositional defiant disorder
	copro/echo and pali phenomena
	stuttering
	drug side effects

are highly threaten school relationships with a risk of isolation for the TS student. Echo and paliphenomena are usually less impairing than coprophenomena, but more than simple tics.

The preoccupation of bothering others often increases tics and causes depressive symptoms i.e. the patient feels as a burden for the others (Marcks et al, 2007). In addition to this, because of tics, TS children could be mocked by the class and labelled with inappropriate nicknames (Wadman et al, 2013; Box 6.1).

Box 6.1   Stereotypical nicknames a TS student may be called.

"Eye guy"
"Upset"
"Annoying"
"Rude"
"Lazy"
"Weird"
"Awkward"
"Alien"

A tic could also be misinterpreted by teachers. The teachers could see it as a disrespectful joke made on purpose by the student to provoke them during lessons. The student may even be punished because of it.

On the contrary, when a TS student is only affected by very mild tics, they will probably not be disturbed by them during school.

ADHD. Even if tics can be more evident than other symptoms, TS behavioural diseases have a higher impact on school, work and social life. Distraction and restlessness at school are often the reason for a first visit.

Moreover, when a TS patient has ADHD, the chances to control tics is lower (Himle & Woods, 2005).

Abwender et al (1996) showed that 56% of TS children having school difficulties were suffering from ADHD, also. ADHD is therefore a predictor of school problems in TS (Figure 6.3).

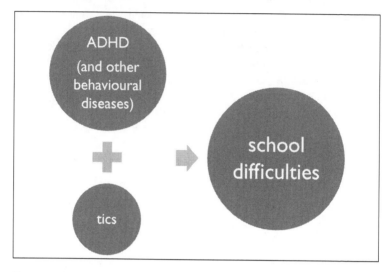

Figure 6.3 School difficulties in TS students are mainly caused by behavioural diseases.

Credit: Cecilia Spalletti.

OC component. When OC component is prevalent in a TS student, usually she will show compulsions that distract her. For example, Kate has the obsession that her TS will cause her school difficulties. During school classes she will be focused on this obsession and therefore she will spend more time in thinking about it rather than achieving any task.

OC component may cause reading problems, as well. For example, when a TS student has these symptoms, the reading could be interrupted and the understanding of the text could be incomplete (e.g. resulting in no memory on part of the text).

Even while writing, OC component may interfere. The compulsion of starting a new line, for example, could make the student lose the sense of the written text. Another example is John's compulsion of deleting any irrelevant typing mistakes: the result will be a ripped piece of paper.

Petra is affected by another OC: symmetry compulsions for books. Until books are in Petra's correct position, she will continue to move them. As a consequence, she won't be able to follow the lesson as she would be too focused on her compulsions.

Mark has, instead, the typical compulsion of checking his school bag. His fear is of leaving some of his school supplies at home. He will be therefore obsessively checking the school bag. Paradoxically, while moving his things in and out of the bag, he will forget something at home.

If the compulsions can't be accomplished, the TS student may have a rage outburst.

N.B. The OC component may regard the relationship with schoolmates (E.g. Matteo strongly demands from Sara to greet him, otherwise he will feel offended and have a rage outburst)! Compulsions/rage outbursts could therefore appear as unjustified for schoolmates, who may consider the TS student as a "weird" or spoilt person. In Chapter 7, other social consequences of OC component are considered.

Learning disorders. Some TS children can have learning disorders. Main manifestations are:

- low grades.
- language difficulties when speaking, writing, reading, listening.
- difficulties with calculations.
- wrong study methods.
- poor skills of organising/summarising information.
- deficit in some memory areas.

TS students often need a tutor at home, and more often, not because of cognitive deficits but because of school phobia or low self-esteem (caused by TS symptoms). Most of the time the tutor is indeed a "presence" during homework, a reassuring figure. Other times, the tutor will help the child with organising the homework agenda or with improving the study method.

School phobia. It can manifest with anxiety and school absenteeism, panic attacks, organic disturbances (e.g. sickness, vomiting, fainting), crying or rage. It usually increases before going to school, while going to school or once the student is at school. The sufferer will typically ask parents to stay at home or to be picked up before the end of the school day (Figure 6.4). The phobia will increase proportionally as the parents adhere to their child's (pathological) requirements. The recommendation for parents is usually to leave the student at school if the symptoms are of a clear anxious origin.

Alert!

Your child has school phobia? Leave them at school when anxiety manifests!

NOSI and oppositional defiant disorder. When TS presents these disorders, the student is seen as "unpleasant" and "awkward", and as a result schoolmates tend to exclude the sufferer from games and conversations. This also happens because these disorders unable the person to follow game and talking rules.

Moreover, TS with oppositional defiant disorder may tend to justify themselves and accuse others. This behaviour also creates a barrier between the TS student and his schoolmates.

Stuttering. It is another symptom which can decrease oral school performances and undermine relationships. Bullying is a common

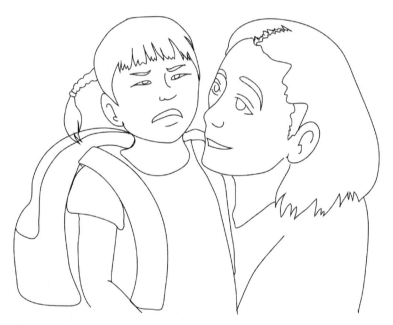

Figure 6.4 A caregiver reinforcing school phobia by picking her child up before school is over.

Credit: Cecilia Spalletti.

result of stuttering. School interventions (see paragraph, "Teachers' experience") may be effective in reducing bullying in classes.

Social anxiety. A high Social Impairment may be accompanied by social anxiety. This type of anxiety may manifest with both avoidant or dependant behaviours within relationships.

Autism spectrum disorders. The social and cognitive deficits of a TS+autism spectrum disorder patient usually requires the presence of a special needs teacher.

Drug side effects. Sleepiness is a frequent drug side effect impairing the TS patient at school. Parents should inform school staff that their son may have side effects from TS drugs (cf. Chapter 4). In this way, teachers will know the reason of his tiredness and will not rebuke him.

Homework time. Caregivers usually struggle to get the child to start homework, and once started, the child has to deal with two major issues: handwriting tics and ADHD. Once home, after a long day at school the student is usually tired and nervous. This is also because of the energy spent at school in controlling symptoms. In his own house – "the safe place" – a child can finally explode with TS symptoms.

Homework is very arduous for TS children, and it usually requires more time than for non-TS students. Because of that, ad hoc recommendations are given to deal with this issue (see Figure 6.5). First, it is better for the child to study by himself. On the other hand, if a patient has a low IQ, or severe tics or psychopathologies, a tutor's/caregiver's help is required. Many parents have stated that it can be difficult to stay with the student while doing homework as he is often "aggressive". For this reason, tutors may be preferred to parents: the unconscious control is higher when in presence of a non-family member (see Figure 6.5).

Secondly, a timetable is often needed to help organising the workload (especially for TS+ADHD students). A complete schedule may include time of beginning and of ending for each subject, and for breaks (Figure 6.5). School subjects may be ordered from the hardest to the less difficult considering age, abilities and preferences, cognitive effort required and urgency for the subject to be ready for exams. A functional way to schedule breaks is to have a short one (e.g. 10 minutes) at the end of each subject or every 45 minutes.

In the following homework schedule (Figure 6.5), Henry must define the start and stop time of each school subject. Finally, he must write down if he has effectively followed the plan or what he otherwise missed.

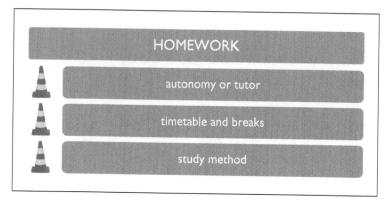

Figure 6.5 Homework's key points for TS students.
Credit: Cecilia Spalletti.

The study method could be an issue as well (Figure 6.5), especially for patients with severe behavioural problems or with learning disorders. Tutors will guide the student towards the improvement of his study method, e.g. by repeating lessons loudly (cf. Table 6.6).

Caregivers and teachers should remember that homework's difficulties are not caused by laziness. We are talking about a disorder! Moreover, symptoms are connected (e.g. Mark's learning difficulties when studying make him more nervous and sad, thus provoking a tic increase). For this reason, the student needs to be helped and not punished!

In conclusion: if the correct therapy and school support are ongoing, the TS student can handle each school-related issue.

Table 6.2 Henry's homework timetable.

Henry's schedule Date: 15th June 2018		Start time	Stop time	Success? If no, note what I have missed.
Subjects (or breaks)	maths	2.30	3.10	√
	break	3.10	3.20	√
	English	3.20	4	√
	break	4	4.10	√
	history	4.10	4.45	stop time 4.40
	break	4.45	4.55	4.40-4.50
	art	4.45	5.30	4.50-5.25

Schoolmates' experience

TS students' Social Impairment is sometimes due to their guilt because of dysfunctional behaviours towards schoolmates. A typical reaction is rage outbursts with verbal or physical aggression (e.g. to yell at schoolmates, to throw others' objects against the wall and break them). Especially when TS has an ADHD or OC component, rage outbursts are frequent and interfere with school relationships (Marcks et al, 2007).

Generally, the presence of a TS student in class affects schoolmates. Even when TS is very mild, they are distracted by the TS student's symptoms during lessons. On the other hand, Jagger et al (1982) highlight that:

- 75% of TS students have been mocked or rejected by schoolmates.
- 25% of TS students have been mocked by teachers and have been more strictly evaluated in exams if compared with schoolmates (as punishment for TS symptoms!).

These attitudes are highly damaging to the vulnerability of the sufferer.

Packer (2005) suggests that TS students' difficulties with classmates are due to (see Figure 6.6): mild bullying (39%), high bullying (28%). On the other hand, 9% is the bullying percentage for a non-TS student (Storch et al, 2007). According to teachers, this difference could be justified by an empathy deficit of TS children (Kadesjö & Gillberg, 2000).

Being bullied triggers two main negative effects for the TS student (Figure 6.7):

- self-esteem decreasing (or further decreasing)
- school avoidances (see Chapter 3) which could evolve in school phobia
    N.B. Avoidances may be the result of severe outbursts with schoolmates (Sukhodolsky et al, 2003).

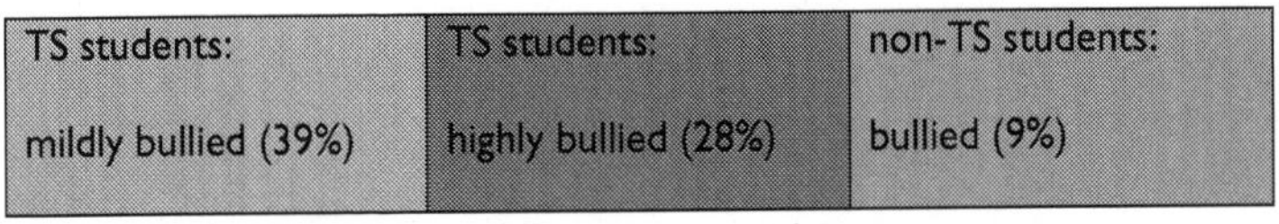

TS students:	TS students:	non-TS students:
mildly bullied (39%)	highly bullied (28%)	bullied (9%)

Figure 6.6 Percentages of TS students being bullied and controls.
Credit: Cecilia Spalletti.

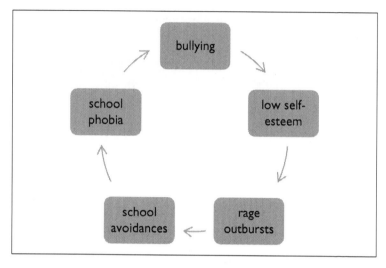

Figure 6.7 Dysfunctional process of being bullied for TS students.
Credit: Cecilia Spalletti.

Before school interventions, schoolmates typically behave in the ways listed here towards a TS student:

- staring at him when tics appear.
- warning him to stop tics.
- miming his tics and behaviours.
- asking him not to disturb the lesson.
- demanding him not to move or to shut up.
- laughing at his school difficulties.
- bullying him with inappropriate nicknames or with tricks.
- isolating him during break time and during gym class.
- excluding him from social events, e.g. birthday parties.

Bullying takes place at school, where the system is often not adequately prepared to protect students, but inevitably occurs also in the extra-scholastic contexts. In these contexts, the protection of parents and school staff is absent, and difficulties could therefore be higher.

Either positive or negative experiences in the childhood of a TS student could have a domino effect on his school life during adolescence, and as a result, during his university or work life (cf.Figure 6.8). Social problems during adulthood may be the result of negative experiences with classmates, peers, and with key educational actors (i.e. parents and teachers) during childhood and adolescence.

Adolescence is, no doubt, the riskier period for negative experiences at school (cf. Figure 6.8). This is because teenagers experience their first social events alone with peers, having only few social skills. Secondly, because of their ongoing body development. They need to accept themselves in a changed body. This is especially harder in case you don't control your movements and sounds!

Tics do not make a difference if the school environment is based on acceptance and cooperation, and when the school itself protects students from bullying. In a "good school" the condition of a TS student usually improves thanks to the relationship with school-mates (see Box 6.2)!

Box. 6.2 Point of view of a comprehensive schoolmate

"It is hard not to notice Sam's tics. At the beginning I was turning my head towards him every time he had a tic. Now, I've learned how to avoid it. If I think about how difficult it was for me not to notice his tics, I understand how difficult it must be for him trying to control them!"

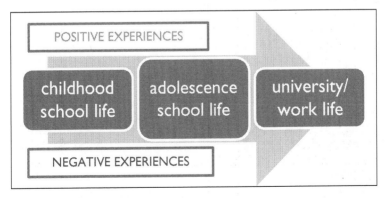

Figure 6.8 The impact of school social life in the future of a TS sufferer.
Credit: Cecilia Spalletti.

Teachers' experience

TS is a complex disease, and it is hard for a teacher to help a sufferer without previous experience of it. For this reason, teachers should be informed by experts about TS features and how to deal with symptoms during school hours (see Table 6.6). For example, teachers should know that:

- tics are neurological, but they may be exacerbated by external conditions such as stress.
- some children with TS can control tics, but only for short periods of time.
- controlling tics requires a high level of effort and may cause attention deficits.
- tics wax-and-wane and vary for typology.

By being made aware of these few points, a teacher can have a better understanding of the syndrome and consequently attempt to create a suitable school environment, based on support and not on judgement or punishment. The child will feel accepted, reduce the negative emotions and, therefore, limit tics (cf. Figure 6.9).

Generally, students consider their teachers, together with parents, as their key adult figures. As a result, the way in which they react towards the TS student is reciprocated by the class. This means that an attitude of openness in a teacher will result in a similar attitude in the whole class. On the contrary, if the child is not welcomed by his key figures, he feels alone and excluded. For instance, if a teacher punishes tics, the student will feel misunderstood and not accepted, which leads his schoolmates to reject him too.

Before exploring experts' intervention at school, we analyse teachers' typical attitudes towards TS students. Rivera-Navarro et al (2014) compare all the stakeholders' (children, parents and teachers) views about TS influence on school (Table 6.3).

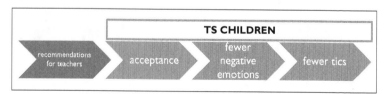

Figure 6.9 The positive process of involving teachers with ad hoc recommendations.

Credit: Cecilia Spalletti.

Table 6.3 Different points of view of the impact of TS on school: children, family, school.

Main TS and school problems, according to . . .

TS STUDENT	PARENTS	TEACHERS
1 relationship with schoolmates and teachers 2 behavioural problems	1 tics 2 relationship with schoolmates and teachers	1 didactic issues

The results of this study highlight how teachers are mainly concerned with difficulties regarding the didactic area. This happens because quite often teachers are not well prepared about the syndrome's social impact. They should know that if a student with TS does not receive the right understanding at school, the risk of Social Impairment increases. In extreme cases, the student will abandon school.

Conversely, the TS student and caregivers are often more informed about TS social issues, and they do their best to prevent negative implications. Usually it is the TS student that focuses more on relationships, whereas parents are too focused on tic control (see Table 6.3). This has a negative influence on the student's acceptance of the syndrome.

To protect TS students from these risks, teachers (and sometimes schoolmates) are trained through informative meetings on the syndrome's features (White et al, 2011). Meetings may be recommended even for mild cases, depending on the family's and clinicians' agreement. Usually meetings are up to 3 or 4 for a student. According to the authors' experience, they should last around 60 minutes for teachers, and around 40 minutes for schoolmates.

N.B. Meetings are often requested by the TS students themselves because of discomfort.

During meetings, participants may be:

- the TS student
- teachers
- TS student's schoolmates and other classmates
- school principal/s
- families

When experts are talking to schoolmates, the TS student can stay outside the classroom if he prefers. This because of the embarrassment of being the centre of attention of the class when talking about his disease. Of course, the TS student's presence at the meeting means that he already accepts – even partially – his condition. Nevertheless, the meeting – also in absence of the TS student – leads to a gradual acceptance of the disease for him. The meeting's aim is for school-mates to be more welcoming with the TS student.

Meetings may be guided by one or more of the following TS experts:

- psychologists
- educators
- doctors
- pedagogues
- actors

Woods et al (2003) demonstrate the efficacy of meetings for teach-ers and schoolmates, especially when a movie on TS (e.g. Gottlieb & Werner, 2008; Figure 6.10) is shown to help the understanding of the syndrome. Informative meetings, with an actor miming a TS person or with the use of comics, also lead to a considerable change in the class group (Marcks et al, 2007). They help explaining to stu-dents the involuntariness (having no negative causes e.g. meanness) of their TS schoolmate's behaviours.

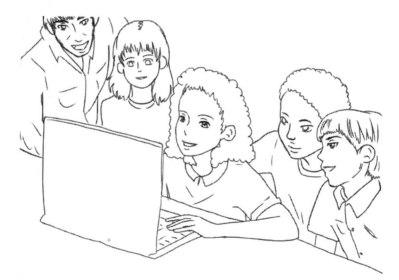

Figure 6.10 Videos are used by experts to explain TS features in schools.
Credit: Cecilia Spalletti.

Encouraging teachers not to underline the appearance of tics, and to apply other case-by-case strategies (see Table 6.6), leads to a considerable improvement in the way a child can live with the syndrome at school.

A common strategy that teachers should adopt to ease TS students is to give them the chance to temporary leave the classroom (see Table 6.6). When tics suddenly explode, causing embarrassment for the student, as well as objective disturbance for the schoolmates, teachers should let the student leave the classroom for a short break. In this way, the student can deal with the tics outside the class. The child can walk in the corridor or go to a designated room to regain the lost control. Once relaxed, the student will be ready to go back to the lesson.

In order to reduce behavioural issues, a special needs teacher can introduce a "token economy" (see Table 6.4). This technique allows the student to control impulsivity. Using this method, the student has to accumulate a sum of tokens for a given number of days in order to win a prize. Tokens are given when the student manages impulsivity. The prize should be decided by the student with the help of a teacher. This is a motivational technique, also used in Parent Training (see Chapter 4 and Chapter 5).

For example, Vanessa is an 8-year-old TS student, and her issue at school is that she can't resist raising her hand. This gesture is distracting the whole class during the lesson and, for this reason her special needs teacher is willing to find a solution. In order to reduce this habit, her teacher creates a weekly token economy. To gain 1 or 2 tokens, Vanessa has the task of avoiding the gesture. She will win 1 token, when she partially resists during the school day; or 2 tokens when she totally resists the impulse. In the case that she can't resist at all, no tokens will be given. If she gains at least 7 tokens in a week (with a maximum of 10 tokens) she will get a given prize, i.e. a box of stickers. In Table 6.4, Vanessa earned 7 tokens, so consequently she will earn the stickers.

Surprisingly, sometimes teachers are more respectful to TS students than their own family are. School can be a safe "place" where a TS person claims their own rights and gains the well-deserved respect for their needs. For example (Figure 6.11), George's teachers invite his family to take him to the doctor for a visit as they noticed that some tics are interfering with his studying. George's family, even knowing about the presence of tics, had waited, without considering any sort of intervention until that moment. Finally, George finds the opportunity to be treated

Table 6.4 Vanessa's token economy table: a technique to limit her impulsivity.

	no resistance	🌀 partial resistance	🌀 🌀 total resistance
Monday			🌀 🌀
Tuesday			🌀 🌀
Wednesday			🌀 🌀
Thursday		🌀	
Friday	---------------		

thanks to his teachers. After a few months of treatment, the family is thankful to George's school.

Creativity in TS patients

One of the abilities that schools should develop in students is creativity. Unfortunately, more often teachers reward students following standard rules as they have to refer to a rigid scholastic system. An example could be one of a teacher who can't reward his student with a high grade for his cute drawing because he didn't follow the instruction of using just black and white markers.

According to Jones' definition (1972), creativity is the combination of flexibility, originality and ability to adopt readily new and unusual cognitive patterns in order to face problems. Creative people have what is called divergent thinking (Guilford, 1956). This way of thinking typically occurs in a free-flowing,

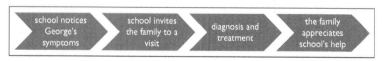

Figure 6.11 A positive cultural process between school, family and healthcare professionals.

Credit: Cecilia Spalletti.

"non-linear" manner, such that many ideas/solutions may be generated in a short time.

Many TS people have a strong talent for arts (especially playing instruments, singing and poetry) and for other activities requiring creativity and divergent thinking (Sacks, 1992). Several famous artists such as Samuel Johnson (Boswell, 1835) and possibly even Mozart were affected by TS (Ashoori & Jankovic, 2007).

Because of their spontaneity, some TS patients are particularly talented in Dionysian arts (cf. Table 6.5) rather than for Apollonian arts (Nietzsche, 1872). Patients with a prevalent OC component may prefer Apollonian style because of their rigour.

Literature underlines that higher dopamine levels and a prevalent use of the right part of the brain (see Figure 6.12), both typical in TS patients (see Chapter 2), correspond to divergent thinking.

Unfortunately, as we said earlier, school often empathises the use of left brain in students. That's the reason why the subject in which TS students are less skilled is usually maths: a subject with less space for creativity.

Recent studies have investigated the specific features of creativity in TS children and adults, also comparing TS people with normal controls (Zanaboni et al, 2011) and with patients affected by other pathologies e.g. Parkinson's disease (Zanaboni et al, 2017).

Results confirm that TS children are around 18% more creative than non-TS children. The main creative feature in TS people, when compared with healthy people, is greater flexibility (i.e. the skills of changing your mind set to overcome a problem).

The study (Zanaboni et al, 2017) compared TS people to people with other disorders and confirmed the TS major predisposition to creativity. It shows TS adults being around 9% more creative than people with Parkinson's disease.

Considering these data in terms of neurotransmitters' functioning, it's not only dopamine that has a role in the development of

Table 6.5 From Nietzsche's art styles to TS patients' talents.

Art style	Apollonian arts	Dionysian arts
Features	Exactness, beauty, symmetry, harmony	Irregular, spontaneous, chaos, emotions, thrill
Example	e.g. architecture	e.g. improvised music

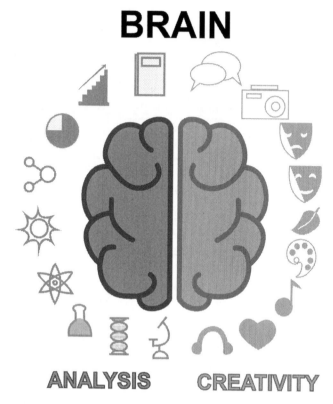

Figure 6.12 Creativity is one expression of the right human brain.
Credit: Cecilia Spalletti.

creativity (and in TS itself), but also others, such as serotonin, are implicated. Furthermore, drugs (e.g. dopaminergic treatments) alter neurotransmitters' action, and therefore creativity levels, as well.

In conclusion, the presence of high levels of dopamine in TS brains doesn't only have the negative impact of causing tics and behavioural symptoms, it also has the positive implication of leading to a divergent thinking. Creative talent may drive TS people to undertake creative school departments/jobs or hobbies (see Chapter 7; Box 6.3). Creativity may therefore help the patient to manage his own syndrome, at school or outside it.

Box 6.3   Pier wrote this song thanks to his strong creativity

A TS child's song: "Don't Change"

Verse 1
Don't cry if you are in trouble,
But like who you are in your heart.
If you are in trap, don't give up.
We are all fantastic,
But with our own defects;
So, never give up.

Verse 2
You are big in my heart.
You can't expect anything better than your best.
A large mountain of memories will never equal a small
Bit of hope.
Never give up.

After school life: working life

As TS may affect the child's educational experience, it can affect their adult work life, too.

It is well-known that at around 18 years of age, a person tends to spontaneously lower his tics, and to manifest mostly, the behavioural aspects of TS. On average, the residual tics are mild and do not undermine any professional placement. On the contrary, behavioural aspects (mostly OC component, SIB and oppositional defiant disorder) sometimes don't allow the employee to obtain a place in whichever business sector he wants, especially those dedicated to public relations.

A study by Palmer & Stern (2015) has investigated whether TS and its comorbidities could hinder the professional achievement. 152 TS adult patients were evaluated. Results showed that severe tics (especially coprophenomena) and associated neurobehavioural pathologies could have a negative impact on work life.

Every employer (or even better every company's doctor) should evaluate the TS features that the worker manifests at that specific moment (see Chapter 3). We talk about "features", and not "symptoms", because positive features, such as creativity (see previous paragraph), may be present as well. Also, a person could decide to benefit from a TS symptom in his work life. For example, a TS patient having mild perfectionism as a comorbidity could opt for a job requiring precision, e.g. working as a bank clerk.

The impact of school and work on Quality of Life has been studied by Shady et al (1995), in a sample of 193 TS adult sufferers. They provided information about:

- academic background (school and university).
- behavioural problems experienced during childhood.
- type of job, and position/role.
- influence of the syndrome on the choice of the job.
- work discriminations related to the syndrome.
- level of job satisfaction.

Data underline three different connections between (see Figure 6.13):
Results suggest that (because of TS):

- 21% of workers are fired.
- 17% of workers are denied a job.
- 12% of workers are denied a promotion.

Assistance is needed, even from law applied to school and work (cf. Chapter 8), in order to protect TS people's rights.

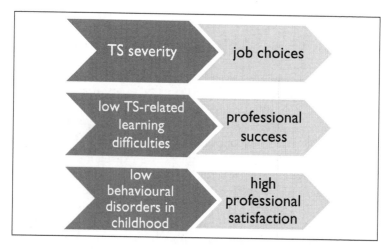

Figure 6.13 Links between TS issues in the course of life and job features.
Credit: Cecilia Spalletti.

Table 6.6 Suggestions for teachers.

N.B. The following suggestions are suitable for the whole school process.
General suggestions

- Ignore tic manifestations. Do not comment on tics, or they will increase.
- Allow the student to leave the class when he feels the need to release tics. If necessary, he can be allowed during exams, as well. N.B. Do not force the student to leave the class, or he may see it as a punishment.
- Choose an adequate desk position for the student. For example, the student may sit close to the door; in this way, he can leave the class without bothering the schoolmates. Another possibility is to leave a place close to the desk (e.g. if the student has the compulsion of touching schoolmates or their objects).
- Allow the student to move in the class, involving him in class activities, such as giving photocopies to each schoolmate.
- Invite the student to a major studying effort during TS remission periods. In this way, he can move forward for the crisis periods.
- Prevent the bullying by watching closely the class' interactions during breaks.
- Ask the family and the student himself if they would like to share the diagnosis with the rest of the class.
- Remember possible side effects of TS medications may occur, e.g. sleepiness.

Ad hoc suggestions

N.B. These suggestions must be evaluated case by case. Please, adopt them only when strictly necessary (during the academic year or during final exams for the sole school subjects in which it is needed). In this way, the student will be challenged as much as possible.

1 Overall effort/slowness (because of tics or other symptoms):

- Scheduling oral exams.
- Limit to one exam a day per subject and if possible, during the first few hours.
- Reducing workload and/or homework (as agreed with the family and tutor).
- Helping the student with checking the diary.
- Suggesting the use of concept maps (on paper or digital) and of a computer with ad hoc software (mother language/foreign language speech synthesis software, tapes with recorded texts, digital dictionary), when at school or at home.

2 Handwriting tics (or other eye/hand tics):

- Reducing the number of questions in written exams. It is better rather than giving extra time, except when written exams can't be reduced (e.g.

(continued)

Table 6.6 (continued)

essays). Actually, TS symptoms are time consuming and cognitive energy decreases over time.
- Using ad hoc software to prevent writing mistakes.
- Give printed written exams.
- Choosing between block letters or italics.

3 Performance or social anxiety:
- (During written exams) giving the first exercise to the student and waiting to give him the following exercise till he has completed the first one.
- Giving the student the possibility to perform exams outside the class. In this way, the student does not feel obliged to control tics and can't bother or be bothered by schoolmates.
- Considering this if reading aloud in front of the class could cause embarrassment. The teacher could also ask the student if they would like to read or not.
- Allowing the student to start with a topic of his own choice during exams.
- Giving the choice of taking part (or not) to school trips such as cinemas, theatres or churches (especially if he suffers from sound tics).

4 Excessive mistakes/slowness in reading and comprehension:
- Favouring oral rather than written exams, with the help of concept maps (on paper or digital).
- Allowing the use of computer with ad hoc software (mother language/ foreign language speech synthesis software, tapes with recorded texts, digital dictionary).
- Reading with the student quizzes of written exams.
- Using simplified exams with multiple choice.
- Considering if reading aloud in front of the class.

5 Difficulties when coordinating writing, reading and listening:
- Considering alternative methods for the dictation, for copying texts or maths problems, for taking notes.
- Allowing the use of a recording device.
- Allowing the use of digital notes.
- Giving a simplified version of listening exams of a foreign language.
- Giving printed written exams.

6 Lack of fluency (because of sound tics or stuttering):
- Focusing on practical skills rather than on knowledges.
- Allowing the use of concept maps (on paper or digital).
- Favouring written exams than oral exams (oral exams can be done outside the class).

7 ADHD and impulsivity:
- Token economy (i.e. reinforcing functional behaviours using a sum of tokens to get a final prize).

Conclusions

School is the gym of life. During these formative years, children should be developing their social and cultural skills, while understanding mutual respect. Being competitive, bullying and neglect work against achieving these goals, and should be remedied by teachers and students, with the help of families when necessary. TS students entering the school environment (and then work life) are burdened with their tics and behavioural problems. They may worry about possible intimidations, being misinterpreted all while having to care about school performances (or work tasks) and therapy-related commitments. The side effects caused by medications could also interfere. Not a simple time for a 6-year-old child or, even worse, for a 13-year-old adolescent! Schools, families and doctors have the complex task of working together to offer the TS child a solid health, education and socialisation.

References

Abwender DA, Como PG, Kurlan R, Parry K, Fett KA, & Cui L. 1996. School problems in Tourette's Syndrome. Vol 53(6). *Archives of Neurology*, 509–511.

Ashoori A, & Jankovic J. 2007. Mozart's movements and behaviour: A case of Tourette's syndrome? Vol. 78. *Journal of Neurol, Neurosurgery, and Psychiatry*, 1171–1175.

Boswell J. 1835. *The Life of Samuel Johnson: Including a Journal of His Tour to the Hebrides, Volume 1*. London, UK, EU: John Murray, 160.

Conelea CA & Woods DW. 2008. The influence of contextual factors on tic expression in Tourette's syndrome: a review. Vol 65(5). *Journal of Psychosomatic Research*, 487–496.

Guilford JP. 1956. The structure of intellect. Vol 53(4). *Psychological Bulletin*, 267–293.

Himle MB, & Woods DW. 2005. An experimental evaluation of tic suppression and the rebound effect. Vol 43(11). *Behaviour Research and Therapy*, 1443–1451.

Jagger J, Prusoff BA, Cohen DJ, Kidd KK, Carbonari CM, & John K. 1982. The epidemiology of Tourette Syndrome: A pilot study. Vol 8. *Schizophrenia Bulletin*, 267–278.

Jones TP. 1972. *Creative Learning in Perspective*. Oxford, UK: John Wiley & Sons, 11–21.

Kadesjö B & Gillberg C. 2000. Tourette's disorder: epidemiology and comorbidity in primary school children. Vol 39(5). *Journal of the American Academy of Child Adolescent Psychiatry*. 548–555.

Marcks BA, Berlin KS, Woods DW, & Hobart Dawies W. 2007. Impact of Tourette Syndrome: a preliminary investigation of the effects of disclosure on peer perceptions and social functioning. Vol 70(1). *Psychiatry: Interpersonal and Biological Processes*, 59–67.

Nietzsche F. 1872. *The Birth of Tragedy from the Spirit of Music.* Leipzig, Germany: E. W. Fritzsch.

Packer LE. 2005. Tic-related school problems: Impact on functioning, accommodations, and interventions. Vol 29(6). *Behavior Modification*, 876–899.

Palmer E & Stern J. 2015. Employment in Tourette syndrome. Vol 86(9). *Journal of Neurology, Neurosurgery, and Psychiatry.* Doi: 10.1136/jnnp-2015-311750.41.

Rivera-Navarro J, Cubo E, & Almazàn J. 2014. The impact of the Tourette Syndrome in the school and the family: perspectives from three stakeholder groups. Vol 36. *International Journal for the Advancement of Counselling*, 96–113.

Sacks O. 1992. Tourette's syndrome and creativity. Vol 305. *BMJ*, 1515.

Seligman MEP. 1972. Learned helplessness. Vol 23. *Annual Review of Medicine*, 407–412.

Shady G, Broder R, Staley D, Furer P, & Brezden P. 1995. Tourette Syndrome and employment: Descriptors, predictors and problems. Vol 19. *PRJ*, 35–42.

Silvestri PR, Baglioni V, Cardona F, & Cavanna AE. 2018. Self-concept and self-esteem in patients with chronic tic disorders: A systematic literature review. Vol 22(5). *European Journal of Paediatric Neurology*, 749–756.

Storch EA, Murphy TK, Chase RM, Keeley M, Goodman WK, Murray M, & Geffken GR. 2007. Peer victimization in youth with Tourette's Syndrome and chronic tic disorder: Relations with tic severity and internalizing symptoms. Vol 29. *Journal of Psychopathology and Behavioral Assessment*, 211–219.

Sukhodolsky DD, Scahill L, Zhang H, Peterson BS, King RA, Lombroso PJ, Katsovich L, Findley D, & Leckman JF. 2003. Disruptive behavior in children with Tourette Syndrome: Association with ADHD comorbidity, tic severity and functional impairment. Vol 42(1). *Journal of the American Academy of Child and Adolescent Psychiatry*, 98–105.

Wadman R, Tischler V, & Jackson GM. 2013. 'Everybody just thinks I'm weird': a qualitative exploration of the psychosocial experiences of adolescents with Tourette syndrome. Vol 39(6). *Child Care Health Development*, 880–886.

Wadman R, Glazebrook C, Beer C, & Jackson GM. 2016. Difficulties experienced by young people with Tourette syndrome in secondary school: a mixed methods description of self, parent and staff perspectives. Vol 16(14). *BMC Psychiatry.* doi: 10.1186/s12888-016-0717-9.

White SW, Sukhodolsky DG, Rains AL, Foster D, McGuire JF, & Scahill L. 2011. Elementary school teachers' knowledge of Tourette

Syndrome, obsessive-compulsive disorder, & attention-deficit/hyperactivity disorder: effects of teacher training. Vol 23. *Journal of Developmental and Physical Disabilities*, 5–14.

Woods DW, Koch M, & Miltenberger RG. 2003. The impact of the tic severity on the effects of peer education about Tourette's Syndrome. Vol 15. *Journal of Developmental and Physical Disabilities*, 67–78.

Zanaboni C. Leckman JF, & Porta M. 2011. Does Tourette Syndrome have a link with creativity? Vol 9. *Yale Child Study Centre Tourette Syndrome Obsessive Compulsive Disorder Research Team Newsletter Yale Bulletin*, 13–16.

Zanaboni Dina C, Porta M, Saleh C, & Servello D. 2017. Creativity assessment in subjects with Tourette Syndrome vs. patients with Parkinson's disease: a preliminary study. Vol 7(7). *Brain Science*, 80.

Chapter 7

Friendship and spare time*

Summary

Tourette syndrome (TS) patients are sensitive subjects; usually they believe in close relationships and establish deep friendships.

Social Impairment, social anxiety and other TS social features influence these relationships, which, therefore, need to be managed by caregivers and specialists.

Friends are another figurative "place", similar to school, where control on TS symptoms improves. When TS children are at school, tic control improves to avoid embarrassment and to fulfil many different commitments; in the same way, when sufferers spend time with friends, tic control is facilitated by emotional wellness.

Spare time (e.g. sports, musical activities, etc.) is important to schedule in order to balance energy expenditure, relaxation and fun. The patient should choose the activities for their spare time, based on the enjoyment they take from those activities. Even during their spare time, the TS patient can take advantage of their high level of creativity.

Introduction

Tourette syndrome sufferers have special needs related to their social life and different attitudes to their pastimes. Some activities and events have a positive impact on tic severity, and when caregivers and patients are aware of this, they mostly select these kinds of experiences. Otherwise, Quality of Life is socially impaired by the syndrome: it is hard for a child to manage the syndrome in social contexts (e.g. in a sport team) and it can be a serious issue for the subject's psychological development, especially when not supported.

* In collaboration with Thomas Spalletti

For this reason, it is relevant to define how to manage spare time and social activities, from a caregiver's and a patient's point of view.

High sensitivity

The TS spectrum includes many personality traits and attitudes: high sensitivity, intelligence and creativity (see Chapter 6) are all relevant elements that, positively or negatively, influence the child's life.

Having a high sensitivity for emotional stimuli (Belluscio et al, 2011; Eddy et al, 2017) can sometimes be an obstacle in facing developmental steps: social and psychological well-being are influenced by this trait (cf. Figure 7.1).

Interacting with others can be a laborious task (Channon et al, 2012), especially when social anxiety or other psychopathological comorbidities are present in TS (Eddy, 2018).

The high sensitivity leads to different results, depending on the support and chances that family and clinicians give the child in understanding, accepting and valuing this quality, by employing it during activities (Figure 7.1). If the innate qualities are supported and cultivated, they can lead to artistic and social skills, and consequently to better self-esteem, self-efficacy and Quality of Life. On the contrary, if they are not used, and therefore not enhanced, the accentuated sensitivity can lead to poor emotional control, low self-esteem and self-efficacy, Social Impairment, and overall to a worse Quality of Life. In order to prevent this, it's fundamental to learn how to pay a particular attention on the emotional life of a child, making sensitivity a powerful resource and not a weak spot.

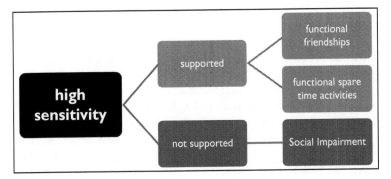

Figure 7.1 High sensitivity: social and psychological consequences.
Credit: Cecilia Spalletti.

Friendship

Friendship represents an important sphere in every phase of the human life (cf. Figure 7.4). Most of TS patients care about it, manifesting a great sensitivity with their peers.

As much as when they are at school (cf. Chapter 6), TS children control their tics when they are with friends. A slight but important difference needs to be stressed. At school, cognitive tasks and embarrassment of showing symptoms to schoolmates are the main elements leading to tic control, which is partially voluntary and involuntary. When with friends, instead, a child feels positive emotions: spending time together (company), being understood (empathy) and sharing a similar point of view (affinity). Thanks to those emotions, tic control takes place. Being an involuntary control, it doesn't steal as many cognitive energies as the ones necessary for the school's conscious control. Given the positive impact of friendships on sufferers' health, caregivers should take it into account when planning their children's spare time.

In other occasions, relationships are complicated to be built for TS sufferers (Albin, 2018). Social skills can be impaired by high sensitivity, by highly socially impairing tics (e.g. coprolalia), or by other TS features (especially social anxiety or OC component).

The main social issue still remains the schoolmates' and teachers' full acceptance of the syndrome (see Chapter 6). A similar situation is seen with out-of-school friends (cf. Box 7.1).

Box 7.1 Alexia's social story brings her to a Tourette Centre

Alexia, a 13-year-old girl, suffered from social exclusion. She used to make 'weird noises'. When tics first started, some neighbourhood friends made fun of her and gave her evil nicknames. They then stopped inviting her to social events. Once, she was the only girl not invited to her friend's pyjama-party, the consequence being spending the whole night crying in her room.

A few days after the party, Alexia decided to go to a Tourette Centre with her parents. From that day on, Alexia has support from doctors and she now knows how to be part of a group!

Social events, like birthday parties, represent a chance to interact with peers and to feel part of a group. Those events have beneficial effects on self-esteem and social skills. As seen in other chapters (e.g. Chapter 6), TS children often experience difficulties because of social stigma: peers (or even other children's parents!) see them as badly behaved children and exclude them from social occasions (Box 7.1). This is a hard experience to accept. Co-protagonists of this exclusion are, at times, the sufferer's parents, scared by the constant mocking of their children and over-worried about the negative effects of their children's Social Impairment. Parents could even prohibit their children to take part into social activities (e.g. sports and summer camps) in order to prevent them from a painful social exclusion. It seems a paradox but this parental attitude offers self-isolation as solution to solve the problem of social isolation: it clearly interferes with the child's social development.

The acceptance of the syndrome is a fundamental step of personal, and therefore, social growth. The first supporting figures in this sense are the parents: when a child is aware of their parents' acceptance of the syndrome, TS will become just an extra feature of life!

Also, it's not rare to see a Tourette's sufferer ending his educational pathway too early (Chapter 6). This decision can lead to many social consequences, as well. When a student quits school, they definitely experience a Social Impairment. On the contrary, participating in school life is a 'gym' of interaction with peers and first friendships. In these cases, parents – being a social model for their children – could prevent social issues at school, for example by organising playdates with schoolmates or meetings between parents at pick up time.

Alert!

An adequate social life is a protection factor against the syndrome severity.

Tics represent the first obstacle in social life because of the marked diversity related to body self-control. Other syndrome-related disorders influence social life, as well (O'Hare et al, 2016).

Social anxiety, OC component and autism spectrum disorders have the following social effects on the sufferer:

Social anxiety and related avoidances (see Chapter 3) interfere when trying to build serene childhood friendships (Erickson, 1950). It is even worse when parents collude with the patient and prevent the child from facing social contexts. Enhancing isolation attitudes has the only outcome of maintaining the sufferer's actual condition (Box 7.2). The child won't gain enough courage to fight the negative circle of low self-esteem and isolation. To stimulate and raise a child, parents' love is certainly fundamental, but often not enough on its own. In the case of social anxiety, caregivers should ask for help to a TS specialist. Psychological support will gradually lead to a deeper understanding for the need of friendships. It will also promote the development of practical social skills, i.e. a pattern of behaviours to functionally interact with others (e.g. how to take part of an ongoing discussion about football within a group of friends).

Box 7.2   The experience of George: social anxiety and psychological support

Parent A.: "George (16 years old) wanted to quit school and his swimming lessons. He was worried about being alone with peers, and he would begin each day whining to the point that we eventually allowed him to stay home. It has been very hard to resist his request, he was really suffering, he wasn't lazy. We realised he was terrified of being surrounded by others. He didn't know what to say, how to simply sit or stand close to others in a room . . .

After two months, my husband and I decided to ask for help. We were referred to a psychologist, and he advised us to send him back to his social contexts. He needed to live a social life in order to stop fearing it. With the specialist's help, George was no longer begging to stay home and we were trying our best to persuade him.

Now our effort is finally visible: he has made some good friends and they are about to organise a weekend trip to the seaside all together".

When TS is comorbid with the *OC component*, social skills may be impaired (Eddy et al, 2017). OC often leads to extreme pickiness when choosing friends, selecting them through pathological criteria. These patients often have a rigorous sense of ethics, which works like a filter in their social life, selecting only the more adequate friends and excluding any other ones (e.g. ethical obsessions strictly define a friend as someone who would never lie).

Alert!

OC component induces extreme social choosiness,

limiting friendships and activities.

TS may in few cases be comorbid with *autism spectrum disorder*. Symptoms include a social functioning deficit. For example, these sufferers often have only one friend, or their social interactions are limited to older or younger people. Activities are usually stereotyped, and games have inflexible rules.

Psychological support helps children, having TS+autism spectrum disorder, in facing these issues. Intervention consists of a social skill training, and in tailored activities that imply social interactions within small and larger groups.

Friendships develop at school, and in other social contexts. In the following paragraph, main social contexts and related leisure activities are analysed, in relation to TS patients' needs.

Spare time, well-being and timetable

Daily activities (including leisure time) exert a great influence on tics and other symptoms, reducing or increasing them, and therefore having an impact on the psychosocial status of the child (see Figure 7.2). Psychosocial well-being, in turn, improves symptoms by reducing Social Impairment. Following this paradigm, a poor psychosocial status with a low quality of spare time activities does not move the sufferer towards wellness.

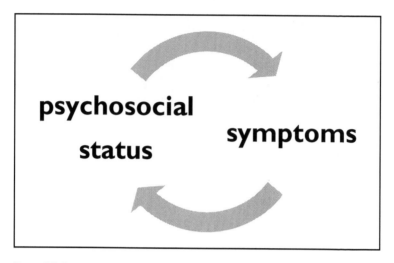

Figure 7.2 Reciprocal relation between psychosocial status and symptoms.
Credit: Cecilia Spalletti.

TS sufferers often show peculiar innate traits (high IQ, creativity and sensitivity), which can be advantageous in specific hobbies. As a result, pathologic manifestations will be modulated.

Personal satisfaction given by spare time activities is a great help for a TS sufferer, it produces a consistent reinforcement of self-esteem, self-efficacy and social skills, leading to a general mood improvement. These activities reduce the effects of various stress factors (including school pressure), which are highly perceived by TS patients (Steinberg et al, 2013).

N.B. In order to generate positive emotions and take benefit from leisure activities, children's choice has to be made on personal interests and passions.

TS diseases may interfere on the constancy of leisure activities, as follows:

• Depressive symptoms (cf. Figure 7.3) lead to lack of motivation in attending assiduously the activities, resulting in a renouncing attitude. This happens as patients don't pay attention to their satisfaction and well-being during and after the activity.

  Patients should be advised by TS specialists and caregivers in reacting against this renouncing attitude: they will finally raise their mood again!

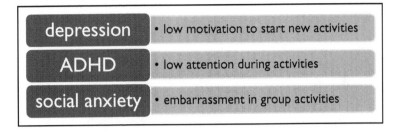

Figure 7.3 TS-related diseases and consequences on spare time activities.
Credit: Cecilia Spalletti.

- ADHD (cf. Figure 7.3). The impulsivity component of ADHD prevents the sufferer to focus on a single activity for the necessary time. Patients usually lose attention and stop the activity. The role of TS specialists and caregivers is again fundamental to reverse the patients' attitude, persuading them on not giving up.
- Social anxiety (cf. Figure 7.3). Group activities imply the closeness to people, often sharing intimate moments; this can be embarrassing (e.g. the feeling of being watched while undressing after a team sport).

To reach biopsychosocial well-being, seven life spheres (see Figure 7.4) should be taken into account. The best evidence of achieving a global well-being is when a person's agenda is covering each sphere. The scheme underlines that relationships (family, friends, partner) have a wider relevance in defining well-being (see previous paragraph, "Friendship" and Chapter 5). School/job, hobbies and sports are daily to weekly (see also Chapter 6), and therefore largely contribute in terms of time. Personal growth and self-care represent a focus on the body and on the psychological care. The devotion to all these areas contributes to the building of a self-equilibrium: the first step for reducing TS symptoms.

An adult's eye is often necessary in the management of time and activities; parents should underline the importance of priorities, when necessary with graphical supports (Figure 7.5).

Once priorities are clear for the child, an efficient resource for a better management of time is to write a schedule, together with the caregiver. The caregiver writes it in agreement with the child; this will give the child a wider sense of responsibility and functional control. N.B. it is especially during the school year that the use of

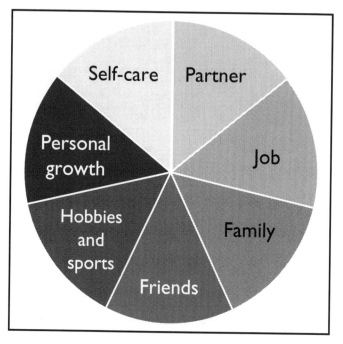

Figure 7.4 Adapted from Strocchi & Jodice (2000): personal life spheres.
Credit: Cecilia Spalletti.

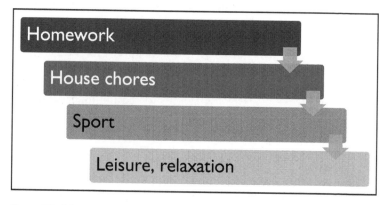

Figure 7.5 A basic priorities' scheme for a child's daily activities.
Credit: Cecilia Spalletti.

Table 7.1 Example of a child's schedule during summer holidays.

	M	T	W	T	F	S	S
9 am–11 am	homework		homework	homework		homework	
11 am–12 am			sport	house chores			house chores
12 am–1 pm	lunch	lunch	lunch	lunch	lunch	lunch	lunch
1 pm–3 pm	leisure	leisure	leisure	leisure	leisure	leisure	leisure
3pm–6 pm	sport				sport		
6pm–7 pm	dinner	dinner	dinner	dinner	dinner	dinner	dinner
7pm–9 pm	leisure	leisure	leisure	leisure	leisure	leisure	leisure

a schedule is suggested. But severe patients benefit from a schedule even during holidays (see Table 7.1). Its use prevents patients from anxiety – and other TS symptoms – generated by sudden activities.

If the caregiver's support in planning the agenda is not sufficient, a psychologist helps the patient in balancing activities of the seven spheres, while also treating tics (see Chapter 4).

Considering hobbies, many lists are diffused worldwide to stimulate patients (cf. Bilsker & Paterson, 2009). In order to improve depressive/anxiety symptoms, the patient is invited by the psychologist to start some hobbies, taken from the list, for a defined period of time; the psychologist will then collect the patient's emotional feedback and underline progress.

Choosing between hobbies, the authors decided to dedicate the following paragraph to sports because of their beneficial impact on tics and other TS features.

Sport

Sport is often a first choice for TS sufferers especially because of their well-known urge to move. Physical activity can help modulating tic frequency and intensity: a significant improvement can be observed during and after sports (Caurín et al, 2014; Nixon et al, 2014). Despite improvement, sport is not considered an official therapy for TS patients!

Another strong advantage of sports is that main TS drugs' side effects (i.e. weight gain and tiredness) (Kim et al, 2018) are reduced by practicing.

Recommendations to set up sport activities

In order to benefit from sports, the TS sufferer should (Kim et al, 2018):

- be consistent with training, i.e. from six weeks upwards.
- start with a less intensive training, and eventually decide if gradually increasing the training.
- reduce training if tics are present/increase. If tics don't decrease, the patient should stop the training.

Sport types

There is no evidence about the direct effect of specific sport types (cf. Table 7.2) on tic modulation. Whereas authors believe the following bullet points can guide the choice between sports (Figure 7.6).

- *Subjective interests* (personal attitudes and passions) make the difference in reducing tics because of the induced self-fulfilment. It should be used as first criterion of choice.
- *Tics' types sometimes influence the choice of a sport.* A tic could directly interfere with a particular sport activity (e.g. Peter's breathing tic prevents him from practicing snorkelling) or it could interfere from a social point of view (e.g. Kate's

Table 7.2 Common types of individual and team sports.

Individual sports	Team sports
tennis	football
swimming pool	volleyball
cycling	basketball
running	hockey
gym	field hockey
martial arts	water polo
ping pong	curling
trekking	handball
skating	rugby
skiing	baseball
climbing	cricket

touching-people tic will lead her to prefer individual sports in order to limit social troubles). N.B. Be aware: patients could opt for extreme/dangerous sports because of their impulsivity! These sports should be avoided as the patients lack self-control. In these cases, other possible activities should be considered.

Alert!

Avoid your child practicing an extreme sport.

- *Sports improve social skills.* Let's see how. Sports imply an acceptance and a conformation to some social rules. Furthermore, being part of a team allows the patient to live a "social modelling" (Bandura, 1971). This means that through observation of other team members' interaction, a person will gradually learn useful skills, increasing his social behavioural repertory.
- *Sports positively hide tics*: this point captures the attention of people with high Social Impairment. E.g. in the swimming-pool a mild breast tic is not visible by others. Another example follows: while cycling, a mild hand tic reduces because of the cyclist holding of the handlebars and, as a consequence, Social Impairment reduces too.

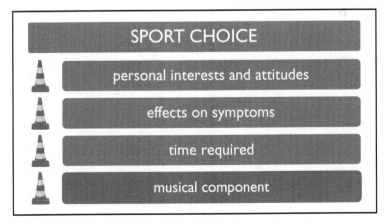

Figure 7.6 Criteria for choosing a sport in TS.
Credit: Cecilia Spalletti.

- *Sports accompanied by music* (e.g. dancing) are preferable because of the positive effect of rhythm on the body movements (see the upcoming paragraph, "Artistic activities").

Agonism

Agonistic sports are not advised in cases of accentuated OC component. Perfectionism and control compulsions can switch the sense of a sport from being a relaxing and pleasant activity into a source of stress and further symptoms. An exaggerated focus on having perfect performances, and on winning, is quite typical for the OC component, and it could lead to frustration in case of failure. For these reasons, before opting to become an athlete, the impact of agonism on the TS sufferer must be considered.

Alert!

Agonism often worsens OC component in TS people.

Agonistic sports are time-consuming (see Figure 7.6), thus taking time away from other activities. Some athletes can dedicate only the weekend to sport activities; for others it is not sufficient. Of course, the beneficial role of a sport must not be an excuse to forget the rest of activities and responsibilities (cf. Figure 7.4 and Figure 7.5). Parents should promise sports as a reward after homework (see "Priorities' scheme"). Also, in adult TS athletes, a caregiver can help the patient in scheduling the weekly sport agenda (cf. Table 7.3).

Table 7.3 A sport schedule helps Brian in reducing tics' and other symptoms' exacerbation.

	M	T	W	T	F	S	S
2–4 pm	basketball			gym	basketball		match
4–6 pm		gym	basketball			gym	
6–8 pm							

Another negative consequence of a strenuous training is an excess of excitement or agitation, which can lead to practise a sport compulsively. This happens especially in patients having an obsession related to their body image. An ad-hoc therapeutic pathway (Chapter 4) is necessary in these cases.

Together with sports, artistic activities represent one of the primary choice for TS patients. The next paragraph informs the reader about the impact of art in Tourette syndrome.

Artistic activities

Many TS patients show a marked creativity (see Chapter 6). This can be channelled into many different activities, leading to a tic reduction (Caurín et al, 2014): e.g. playing an instrument, singing and dancing.

TS patients seem to favour music-related activities above other artistic activities. Musical rhythm affects tics, as it follows (Scataglini et al, 2017): tics are arrhythmic movements, conflicting with music rhythm. Passive (e.g. listening to a song) and active (e.g. playing guitar) participation to music activities is effectively able to reduce tic frequency (Bodeck et al, 2015).

Even artistic activities not involving body or music – such as painting – can improve symptoms and psychosocial well-being. Promoting these activities, especially in cases with high artistic abilities, will help cultivating inclinations. A child will increase their self-esteem and will finally perceives themself as competent in the chosen activity.

Despite the great possibility to express their talent in artistic activities, TS patients often struggle in adapting to the task-related and its social rules. Considering the two different approaches to arts – Dionysian and Apollonian (see the paragraph, "Creativity in TS patients", Chapter 6) – authors recall the prevalence of the Dionysian approach in TS patients. TS impulsive traits complicate the submission to standard methods. When the patient finally successes in the adaptation to rules, his involvement in the artistic activity has a double positive effect: tic reduction and socialisation.

Nowadays art is becoming more and more technologic, and caregivers frequently ask clinicians how to handle electronic devices. TS Centres' experience of this topic is reported in the next paragraph.

Electronic devices

In the last two decades, electronic devices have been taking over our lives. TS patients need special care regarding activities based on the use of technology as it can increase tics (Himle et al, 2014). Children and adolescents' hobbies often involve the use of technology (e.g. game console, television, smartphone, computer and tablet). Parental intervention is necessary to avoid over-use. When the caregiver's help is not sufficient, a TS specialist should be contacted.

- Video gaming requires a huge cognitive effort, and a prolonged use can be a source of distress and overexcitation, increasing TS symptoms (Caurín et al, 2014). Time management and supervision (i.e. playtime should be short and scheduled) help children to dedicating time to these pleasant activities, avoiding negative effects. The author (CZD) advices a maximum of an hour per day of video gaming. Parents can easily identify the best time to game during the day, based on child's reactions (e.g. bedtime is usually the least favourable). Once again, the entertainment should come after duties. Daytime – after homework – is, therefore, the best time option to use devices.

  A peculiar class of videogames requires the use of the whole body to play ("full-body video games"): physical exercise will be added to the cognitive one. As for any other physical activity, a benefit can be observed in motor symptoms (see studies on ADHD by Weerdmeester et al, 2016), but an excessive use exacerbates them. The high attractiveness of full-body video games could have the power to "pick up" a depressed sedentary youth, promoting physical activity and affecting the mood.

- Watching television is another activity that needs to be monitored as it increases tics (Caurín et al, 2014), consequently its use can't exceed. Cognitive passive tasks -including TV- produce distress if prolonged during the day. If playing video games requires a direct participation and produce an outburst of energy (e.g. tapping on the commander), watching TV is a passive activity in which the brain receives inputs, but doesn't produce enough outputs. Accumulated tension from these inputs must be expressed, and tics represent an easy way of expression. Television is a tic trigger especially when programmes are not of the sufferer's interest, or when it is watched for too long and attention declines.

- Social networking and chatting are hard activities to limit in adolescents and adults. Specialists advice the use of a software that set a time limit on usage. An excess could conduct to social problems, such as oppressing a friend or partner. A regular use of these instruments should represent a secondary communication channel, which cannot substitute the primary one: face-to-face interactions.
- Web surfing must be monitored, as well, because of the high risk for patients of becoming compulsive (see studies on ADHD by Weinstein et al, 2015; see also Internet addiction, compulsive buying online and pathological gambling in Chapter 3). Caregivers should not adhere to the increasing requests of the patient related to the use of web devices. Furthermore, credit cards shouldn't be left with minors in order to prevent extra purchasing.

Conclusions

This chapter's intent is to move patients' and caregivers' attention from duties to leisure, in a therapeutic and over-therapeutic sense. Positive effects will be directly influencing the mood of the sufferer, and in second line also his tics. The authors have chosen not to consider religious activities and religious groups because of the vastness of the topic, and for ethical reasons.

The suggested lifestyle is based on global (i.e. biopsychosocial) wellness, following the main principles of the World Health Organization (2014).

References

Albin RL. 2018. Tourette syndrome: A disorder of the social decision-making network. Vol 141(2). *Brain*, 332–347.

Bandura A. 1971. *Social Learning Theory*. New York, NY, USA: General Learning Press, 10–16.

Belluscio BA, Jin L, Watters V, Lee TH, & Hallett M. 2011. Sensory sensitivity to external stimuli in Tourette syndrome patients. Vol 26(14). *Movement Disorders*, 2538–2543.

Bilsker D & Paterson R. 2009. *The Antidepressant Skills Workbook*. Vancouver, BC, Canada: Centre for Applied Research in Mental Health and Addiction (CARMHA) and BC Mental Health & Addiction Services (BCMHAS), 18–29.

Bodeck S, Lappe C, & Evers S. 2015. Tic-reducing effects of music in patients with Tourette's syndrome: Self-reported and objective analysis. Vol 352(1–2). *Journal Neurological Science*, 41–47.

Caurín B, Serrano M, Fernández-Alvarez E, Campistol J, & Pérez-Dueñas B. 2014. Environmental circumstances influencing tic expression in children. Vol 18(2). *European Journal Paediatric Neurology*, 157–162.

Channon S, Drury H, Gafson L, Stern J, & Robertson MM. 2012. Judgements of social inappropriateness in adults with Tourette's syndrome. Vol 17(3). *Cognitive Neuropsychiatry*, 246–261.

Eddy CM, Cavanna AE, & Hansen PC. 2017. Empathy and aversion: the neural signature of mentalizing in Tourette syndrome. Vol 47(3). *Psychological Medicine*, 507–517.

Eddy CM. 2018. Social cognition and self-other distinctions in neuropsychiatry: Insights from schizophrenia and Tourette syndrome. Vol 82. *Progress in Neuro-psychopharmacology and Biological Psychiatry*, 69–85.

Erickson H. 1950. *Childhood and Society*. New York, NY, USA: W.W. Norton & Co, 21–47.

Himle MB, Capriotti MR, Hayes LP, Ramanujam K, Scahill L, Sukhodolsky DG, . . . , & John Piacentini. 2014. Variables Associated with Tic Exacerbation in Children with Chronic Tic Disorders. Vol 38(2). *Behavior Modification*, 163–183.

Kim DD, Warburton DER, Wu N, Barr AM, Honer WG, & Procyshyn RM. 2018. Effects of physical activity on the symptoms of Tourette syndrome: A systematic review. Vol 48. *European Psychiatry*, 13–19.

Nixon E, Glazebrook C, Hollis C, & Jackson GM. 2014. Reduced tic symptomatology in Tourette syndrome after an acute bout of exercise: An observational study. Vol 38(2). *Behavior Modification*, 235–263.

O'Hare D, Helmes E, Eapen V, Grove R, McBain K, & Reece J. 2016. The impact of tic severity, comorbidity and peer attachment on Quality of Life outcomes and functioning in Tourette's syndrome: Parental perspectives. Vol 47(4). *Child Psychiatry & Human Development*, 563–573.

Scataglini S, Andreoni G, Fusca M, & Porta M. 2017. Effect of rhythmic music auditory stimulation on tics modulation in Tourette syndrome: A case study. Vol 5(5). *Open Access Journal of Neurology & Neurosurgery*, 555673. doi: 10.19080/OAJNN.2017.05.555673.

Steinberg T, Shmuel-Baruch S, Horesh N, & Apter A. 2013. Life events and Tourette syndrome. Vol 54(5). *Comprehensive Psychiatry*, 467–473.

Strocchi MC & Jodice L. 2000. *La coppia che non scoppia: Educazione sentimentale*. Verona, IT, EU: Positive Press, 1–172.

Weerdmeester J, Cima M, Granic I, Hashemian Y, & Gotsis M. 2016. A feasibility study on the effectiveness of a full-body body videogame intervention for decreasing Attention Deficit Hyperactivity Disorder symptoms. Vol 5(4). *Games Health Journal*, 258–269.

Weinstein A, Yaacov Y, Manning M, Danon P, & Weizman A. 2015. Internet addiction and Attention Deficit Hyperactivity Disorder among schoolchildren. Vol 17(12). *Israel Medical Association Journal*, 731–734.

World Health Organization. *Twelfth General Programme of Work 2014-2019. Not merely the absence of disease.* 2014. Ginevra, CH, EU: World Health Organization, 18.

Chapter 8

Tourette syndrome and the law*

Summary

The neurological nature of TS needs to be stressed when evaluating patients' imputability in committing illegal acts. In addition, late diagnosis and treatment can have a devastating impact on the legal (besides the social) life of patients with TS. The aim of this chapter is to inform caregivers about the legal implications of TS features; each country has its own medico-legal settlements. Beyond tics, patients' psychosocial "fragility" increases their likelihood of involvement in legal matters. Cases of patients, caregivers and doctors facing legal TS-related problems have been reported. TS is not taken into adequate consideration by justice and society; investigating and raising awareness in this field is necessary.

Introduction

Every sufferer has the benefit of rights, and society is the place where he can find support to preserve them. These rights can be divided into four areas, namely health care, education, work and family (Figure 8.1). With health care, the authors refer to the holistic biopsychosocial wellness' paradigm (World Health Organization, 2014). It is the role of justice to guarantee the social order through citizens' (TS citizens included) adherence to the law. On the other hand, TS people should trust justice and rely on it, either when demanding their own rights to be respected or when they break the rules. In this chapter, the role of the law in relation to Tourette syndrome is introduced to the reader from a medico-legal point of view, without referring to the complexity of country-by-country legislations.

---

* In collaboration with Selenia Greco

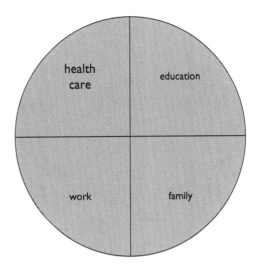

Figure 8.1 The sufferer's rights.
Credit: Cecilia Spalletti.

The syndrome can impact patients' lives from a legal point of view, involving them in civil (i.e. disputes between individuals or other private parties, e.g. malpractice) and criminal (i.e. offences against the state or the government, e.g. theft) matters; families and social contexts are also implicated. In a few severe cases – according to local legislation – TS patients benefit from disability facilitations such as exemptions for drugs costs. In the majority of cases though, social and legal advantages are still not guaranteed to patients and having a disability label represents an obstacle to TS patients' freedom (see denial of driving licence and other examples in the next paragraph).

Alert!

Report inflicted injustices to your TS team and to local authorities. Knowledge about TS rights will increase.

The main syndrome's feature to deal with in legal context is impulsivity (see Ch. 3). All TS symptoms include this issue, which limits patients' possibilities of acting thoughtfully. It also explains a peculiar TS inclination towards bad companies, risky and unlawful conducts (Jankovic et al, 2006).

This overview on legal aspects regarding the syndrome provides an introduction to the patient's imputability, and implications for main stakeholders (patients, caregivers and doctors).

Imputability is described according to Italian law; country-by-country differences may exist.

The imputability (i.e. the legal term for responsibility of one's action, which allows the applicability of penalties) is accorded when, at the moment of the unlawful act, the patient has both the:

1   capacity to understand
2   capacity to take action

The first refers to the possibility of the patient to understand reality, including the presence of his symptoms. In TS people this is present, albeit it can be slightly delayed (Moretto et al, 2011).

The second means the capability to act according to the patient's intention. In TS, this is present in some occasions, and absent in some other ones (Cavanna & Nani, 2013), with no differences considering age (Ganos et al, 2015). Differently, in full mental disorders (e.g. schizophrenia) both capacities are absent. As seen in Chapter 2, Jankovic (1997) explains that tics can be unvoluntary, involuntary or automatic: tics are therefore considered half-voluntary. Behavioural diseases are mostly outside the control of the patient, and therefore involuntary. Ergo, TS is a neurological syndrome having psychological components (see also Chapter 2).

The problem is that courts are not aware of TS, or, even worse, don't accept its double nature! Judges frequently interpret TS symptoms as psychological or neurologic, or non-pathologic, ending the trial with negative outcomes for the patient.

- If TS is seen as psychological only, the patient will be treated as a person suffering from mental illness. He will be sent to psychiatric facilities, and therefore deprived of his freedom, meaning a correct healthcare, closeness to his family and/or an employment (cf. Figure 8.1).
- If the pathology is seen as neurological only, the patient will be considered not responsible for tics, and responsible for his behavioural conducts. He can, as a consequence, be unjustly condemned, thus losing his sufferer's rights when serving his sentence.

- If TS has never been diagnosed or it is denied by the judge, the patient will be processed as a healthy citizen, with total responsibility of his actions. He will be condemned for his own symptoms, and therefore his global rights will be limited.

The court is in charge of judging if a TS subject had the ability to take action or not (the ability to understand is usually maintained) in the exact moment of the outlawed act. Usually, expert TS doctors help the court in this task. Considering the ability to take action during the act, three possibilities can occur (Table 8.1).

In case it is present, the person is imputable. If it is absent, the person is not imputable. It can happen that the person has a partial ability to take action (or to have it for an action and not the another one), and in this case he would be assigned a partial penalty.

In order to clarify intentionality, doctors and the court also analyse the benefits that the patient can obtain through the unlawful act. A sufferer could profit from the disease and mime a symptom with the goal of obtaining money or other advantages, such as work subsidies or invalid badges for parking. In this case, the capacity to take action is present in that moment and the patient is imputable.

Alert!

The scientific community needs to develop a consensus on TS expertise certification for clinicians.

Table 8.1 The TS patient's imputability in relation to his ability to take action.

Ability to take action	Imputability
present	yes
absent	no
partial	partial

The difficulty of defining the imputability of patients underlines once more the necessity for a TS expert clinicians' certification.

Patients and the law

The first stakeholder in law issues is clearly the patient. Each symptom has a peculiar impact. In this paragraph, the primary analysis is dedicated to tics, and secondly, behavioural issues are examined.

The most invalidating tics for legal aspects are:

- shouting tic.
- the repetition of blasphemies and swear words (cf. coprolalia's definition in Chapter 3).
- lewd gesture (cf. copropraxia's definition in Chapter 3).
- touching others' genitals.
- the repetition of others' words (cf. echolalia's definition in Chapter 3).
- the repetition of others' gestures (cf. echopraxia's definition in Chapter 3).
- inconvenient utterance/gesture in public places (cf. NOSI's definition in Chapter 3).
- self-harming (cf. SIB in Chapter 3).

These symptoms can bother or frighten the closest people (see Figure 8.2), such as neighbours if the patient is at home, schoolmates at school, colleagues at work or fellow-citizens in public spaces (e.g. on public transport or at the church). Vice versa, family and friends are usually informed about symptoms and don't react with fear; they are sometimes annoyed by these issues but mostly struggle for the defence of the sufferer's rights.

Tics and behavioural issues lead to the following legal (civil and criminal) and social consequences (Gullucayir et al, 2009; Porta et al, 2018):

- a fine (e.g. Ron gets a fine because of his sound tics violating the condominium's rules).
- police intervention (e.g. a bank clerk calls it, assuming the TS patient is a substance abuser).
- being bullied, school remark or suspension (see also Chapter 6).
- work deskilling/harassment/dismissal (e.g. Tom's boss moves him to the shop's back office to prevent customers from noticing his tics).

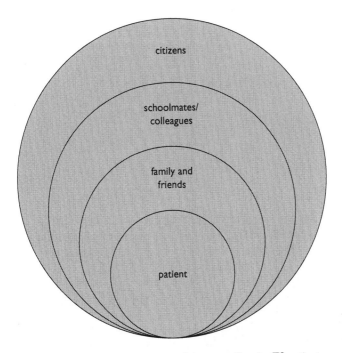

Figure 8.2 Social life contexts: people surrounding the TS patient.
Credit: Cecilia Spalletti.

- social exclusion (e.g. the chorus excludes Johnny because of his sound tics).
- arrest (e.g. Emma's motor tics are misinterpreted on the bus, causing her to be arrested for assaulting a ticket inspector).
- hospitalisation, including compulsory psychiatric treatment.
- driving licence denied.
- military service rejection.
- gun licence denied.

These outcomes are often worse than symptoms themselves, and they may cause further health problems. In order to limit these consequences, European and American countries are distributing a TS identification card to be displayed in social/legal contexts (Figure 8.3).

Tics are accompanied by behavioural symptoms, being often more socially impairing because of their complex mechanism. The most invalidating ones for legal aspects are the most externalised, namely:

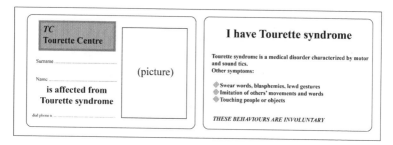

Figure 8.3 Facsimile of a TS identification card.
Credit: Cecilia Spalletti.

- compulsions (e.g. stalking schoolmates for homework).
- oppositional defiant disorder (e.g. parroting a train passenger).
- rage/aggression (e.g. cruelty towards animals at the park).
- addiction (e.g. smoking in prohibited areas, such as inside hospitals).
- personality disorders (e.g. inconsistent behaviours with colleagues).

Consequences are the same as for tics (see the earlier bullet list), but usually, behavioural symptoms are too complicated to be identified as a pathologic condition by fellow-citizens, including the court. Tics are visible and/or audible and, therefore, more often they bother people surrounding the patient, whereas behavioural issues are subtle and less detectable. Behavioural problems are generally the most legally invalidating TS symptoms.

Recently (Porta et al, 2018), four adult OCTD patients (Dell'Osso et al, 2017) with legal injunctions for their TS, have been described. Two of them were bullied because of their syndrome during adolescence, and they were diagnosed and treated only as adults. Their main issues were prison sentences, psychiatric detention and work dismissal. The authors speculate a link between being bullied in childhood and social/legal issues in adulthood (see also Billstedt et al, 2017), especially when late diagnostic-therapeutic pathway is concomitant (Mol Debes et al, 2008).

Alert!

Being bullied for TS can be a predictor for social/legal issues in adulthood. Ask for early psychological support.

Caregivers and the law

Caregivers (parents, partners, siblings, teachers, educators, bosses, coaches and others) could be stakeholders in law issues, especially when having legal responsibility towards minors. The main consequences are listed here:

- restrictions of parental/matrimonial rights (e.g. a two-sibling family needed to be separated because of severe obsessions of the sufferer towards the other sibling).
- caregivers' indictment for children's acts (e.g. an educator was accused because he didn't inform parents of their daughter's self-harming while under his protection).
- work absenteeism because of the sufferer's medical visits (cf. Tourette Centres are still few and sometimes far away from families).
- economic debts caused by the patient's symptoms (e.g. gambling, hoarding) or drug costs.
- sentences for not recognising the patient's syndrome (e.g. a teacher was accused for asking a child with coprolalia to wash his mouth with soap). Caregivers sometimes justify the patient's non-symptomatic actions because of having behavioural problems themselves.

Box 8.1   Example of caregivers' involvement in a TS patient's penal act

In 2017 Tom – a 14 year old, living in a big town of southern Italy – and his parents were accused of having set fire to a neighbours' house. Tom suffers from TS, including a severe obsession towards his neighbours. The judge called Tom's doctor for a consultation. Finally, Tom and his parents were acquitted because he was considered as without ability to take action during the act; his parents tried their best to limit the act, then called the police.

The selection of such a severe clinical case (Box. 8.1) has the only intent of stimulating caregivers' protection of family's rights.

Doctors and the law

TS doctors could also be stakeholders by incurring in legal issues. They have the duty to work in team (Chapter 3) and follow the gradual algorithm of the official treatment guidelines (see Chapter 4). Whereas the latter are often unknown, inapplicable or not followed.

The administration of TS drugs and their side effects could also lead the doctor to such problems. Doctors must inform TS families about the existence of TS approved and off-label drugs and their side effects and ask for patients'/caregivers' consent before prescribing them. Minors' assent is also required in many countries.

Reimbursement for inefficacy of treatments – namely drugs, HRT and DBS (cf. Chapter 4) – is another common economic-legal issue. It is sometimes the patients asking for it because they are not satisfied of results. In some cases, this discontent derives from patients' unrealistic expectations about therapies.

Examples of doctors' engagement in lawsuits are:

- John, a 30-year-old man, accused his doctor after suffering sexual side effects of drugs and for having been left by his wife.
- Eveline, a famous model, indicted her neurologist for losing her job. She had gained weight by drugs assumption, without having been informed about the possible side effects.
- Tim's parents asked his psychoanalyst for a reimbursement of the three-year-long psychoanalysis because tics didn't improve. (HRT, together with other CBT techniques, is the only official psychological intervention for TS).

    Patients' and caregivers' *low compliance* in following doctors' prescriptions can have legal consequences for:
- patients, e.g. John was sentenced as he had a car accident while driving without taking his medications.
- caregivers, e.g. a mum was accused for increasing her son's drug dosage causing him irreversible harm.
- doctors, e.g. an inpatient unit was indicted for a TS sufferer who committed a crime on the day he left the hospital without permission.

Privacy is another matter that can involve legal repercussions for the three stakeholders. The authors have decided not to expand the topic because it is beyond the scope of this chapter.

In literature, only a few papers have been published about TS and the law (Jankovic et al, 2006), thus, leading to a lack of legal prevention offered to families, and to a poor understanding of TS at courts. Nowadays Tourette syndrome patients, caregivers and doctors can't yet be properly defended by justice.

Conclusions

Early diagnosis and therapy prevents patients and families from high Social Impairment and from legal issues. Because of its social implications, Tourette syndrome can't be treated only from a clinical point of view. In order to guarantee a complete case management, Tourette Centres' clinicians need to co-work with all local stakeholders: caregivers, school/workplace staff, social workers, law professionals and TS associations. The latter are active worldwide in spreading information and defending patients; in the last decades, internet-based support is facilitating this global intervention. The final goal is educating citizens to respect TS patients' personal and social rights, and therefore improving the TS community's Quality of Life.

References

Billstedt E, Anckarsäter H, Wallinius M, & Hofvander B. 2017. Neurodevelopmental disorders in young violent offenders: Overlap and background characteristics. Vol 252. *Psychiatry Research*, 234–241.

Cavanna AE & Nani A. 2013. Tourette syndrome and consciousness of action. *Tremor and Other Hyperkinetic Movements (New York, N.Y.)*, 3. tre-03-181-4368-1. doi:10.7916/D8PV6J33.

Dell'Osso B, Marazziti D, Albert U, Pallanti S, Gambini O, Tundo A, . . . , & Porta M. 2017. Parsing the phenotype of obsessive-compulsive tic disorder (OCTD): A multidisciplinary consensus. Vol 21(2). *International Journal of Psychiatry in Clinical Practice*, 156–159.

Ganos C, Asmuss L, Bongert J, Brandt V, Münchau A, & Haggard P. 2015. Volitional action as perceptual detection: Predictors of conscious intention in adolescents with tic disorders. Vol 64. *Cortex*, 47–54.

Gullucayir S, Asirdizer M, Yavuz MS, Zeyfeoglu Y, & Ulucay T. 2009. Criminal and legal responsibilities in Tourette's syndrome. Vol 46. *The Israel Journal of Psychiatry and Related Sciences*, 221–225.

Jankovic J. 1997. Tourette syndrome. Phenomenology and classification of tics. Vol 15(2). *Neurologic Clinics*, 267–275. Review.

Jankovic J, Kwak C, & Frankoff R. 2006. Tourette's syndrome and the law. Vol 18. *Journal of Neuropsychiatry and Clinical Neuroscience*, 86–95.

Mol Debes NM, Hjalgrim H, & Skov L. 2008. Limited knowledge of Tourette syndrome causes delay in diagnosis. Vol 39. *Neuropediatrics*, 101–105.

Moretto G, Schwingenschuh P, Katschnig P, Bhatia KP, & Haggard P. 2011. Delayed experience of volition in Gilles de la Tourette syndrome. Vol 82. *Journal of Neurology, Neurosurgery, and Psychiatry*, 1324–1327.

Porta M, Servello D, Dell'Osso B, Zanaboni Dina C, Bona A, & Alleva GC. 2018. Critical aspects in the legal defence of patients with Tourette's Syndrome: An Italian case series. Vol 61. *International Journal of Law and Psychiatry*, 1–5.

World Health Organization. Twelfth General Programme of Work 2014–2019. Not merely the absence of disease. 2014. Ginevra, CH, EU: World Health Organization, 17–22.

Chapter 9

Giuseppe and his coughing OCTD*

Summary

Giuseppe is a boy with Tourette syndrome (TS) – subtype OCTD. His main symptom was coughing, which didn't allow him to attend school anymore. After several improper diagnoses and treatments, which didn't solve the problem, he was finally managed by a TS team: the diagnosis was clarified, and a combined treatment of drugs and psychological interventions was prescribed. The psychological intervention included Habit Reversal Training (HRT), Parent Training and school meetings. Giuseppe recovered when he was 17, after 3 years of therapy. Now he attends school with no coughing or other disturbances: his Quality of Life has been restored.

Introduction

A clinical case is the best way to practice all the knowledge learned and given recommendations related to a specific disease. Giuseppe's history was chosen because, being a teenager, he had lived with 17 years of TS and he finally overcame the worst period with the syndrome, i.e. adolescence (Robertson et al, 2017). Treatment has been adapted to take into account the natural history of the disorder (Leckman, 2003), and it has also been tailor-made based on Giuseppe's subjectivity. His experience underlines the importance of family and social contexts (e.g. school) in approaching tics, the OC component and comorbid symptoms (Verdellen et al, 2011; Dell'Osso et al, 2017). The focus is on describing the phases and techniques of his psychological intervention.

---

* In collaboration with Davide Dèttore, Donatella Comasini and Roberta Galentino

The case

Giuseppe – then 15 years old – arrived, together with his parents, for a first neurological visit to Milan Tourette Syndrome Centre in April 2015. The reason for the visit was a very intense cough, which started 11 months before, preventing Giuseppe from going to school. The cough was not present during the rest of the day. From the age of 6, Giuseppe had different types of motor and sound tics that didn't cause him any trouble. Because of that, the family didn't previously ask for any visits with a specialist.

After the family doctor and the otolaryngologist excluded other organic pathologies and after many therapeutic attempts with insufficient results, Giuseppe was referred to the local Child Neuropsychiatric Centre where he started pharmacological treatments for TS, without success. This is how Giuseppe's diagnostic-therapeutic pathway at Milan TS Centre began.

Alert!

TS patients need to be followed by a TS team.

Anamnesis

Giuseppe was born on the 1st of April 2000 in Trento, a town in northern Italy, where he lives with his parents and brother Nicola (an 11-year-old boy) and attends the second year of High School. Giuseppe is from a wealthy family: his father, a 55-year-old vet, and his mother, a 53-year-old dentist, are very focused on their careers and quite unaffectionate (Pozza et al, 2015). During the first meeting, the non-verbal communication of the parents is poor. They can't maintain eye contact, the facial expression is static, and the interpersonal space towards the clinicians and their son too large. The parents are also denying any psychodiagnostic hypothesis speculated by the doctor regarding their son's issues. For this reason, they favour the Neurology Department (where Milan TS Centre is located) over Child Neuropsychiatry. During the first clinical interview with the parents, the TS team – consisting of a neurologist, a psychologist and a psychotherapist – detects a bilinear familiarity (mother with OC component traits and father with severe OCTD).

Giuseppe is smart, "adultified" and hyper-responsible. Since his childhood he has been spending most of his time studying and getting great school results. He only has a couple of friends, without any close relationships. He has a good relationship with his brother Nicola, a healthy young boy.

His after-school activities are athletics, on an agonistic level, and piano. Giuseppe shows very high musical ability, a typical feature for TS (see Chapter 6).

Because of the symptoms manifested at school, Giuseppe's family opts for a variety of solutions to prevent his studies from being interrupted. During his first year at high school, Giuseppe has a tailor-made schedule because of his insistent coughing tic. During his second year, he has to be home schooled. Even this last solution doesn't prove to be efficient as any contact with school-related stimuli (even just a book) triggers a severe coughing bout despite being at home. Later on, the symptoms extend to sport hours, especially at the end of training sessions or competitions, even though the cough is less violent when compared to attacks related to school stimuli.

On January 2016, Giuseppe has to give up studying, even from home (Allen et al, 2018). From this moment on, given the high Social Impairment, Giuseppe asks his parents to talk to a specialist. Classmate support is poor and often turns into mocking rather than helping. The teachers, having no experience of managing a TS student, find it difficult to face the situation, and as a consequence, react to it. Ensuring that Giuseppe keeps up to date with his homework, oral and written tests, they, unknowingly, negatively impact on the student's clinical condition. The parents, on the other hand, are afraid of their child missing a year of school and therefore cause him greater stress when continuously asking to try to attend.

Alert!

In case of a child's school disease, do not follow your instinct, but ask for a psychological consultation.

Neuropsychological assessment

Giuseppe is invited for the neuropsychological assessment at Milan TS Centre. Giuseppe's parents deny the problem, showing mistrust towards the psychological approach (Gava et al, 2007). However, during the treatment, the team has the opportunity of increasing the whole family's compliance, involving everyone in the meetings.

During the visit, Giuseppe manifests a typical oppositional defiant attitude (cf. Chapter 3), challenging doctors and parents and not answering when asked, but expressing sadness on his face. The team carries out two assessment sessions with Giuseppe and his parents. Together with a detailed clinical interview, the following scales are used:

- The Children's Yale-Brown Obsessive-Compulsive Scale – CY-BOCS (Scahill et al, 1997) underlines obsessions related to contamination (animals and objects contaminated with dirt and germs that Giuseppe might touch), order and symmetry, excessive worries towards body parts (e.g. chest). Giuseppe has compulsions regarding hygiene (cleaning his hands excessively), control, calculation (in particular counting notes when he is playing the piano), order, symmetry and eating rituals. The predominant symptomatology is the coughing (both tics and OC component), triggered by school anxiety.

    The compulsive component (CY-BOCS 15/20) is more severe than the obsessive one (CY-BOCS 10/20): the total being 25/40 with avoidances and caregivers' involvement in rituals.
- The Yale Global Tic Severity Scale – YGTSS (Leckman et al, 1989) evidences different typologies of motor and sound tics for a total resulting in 60%, with a Social Impairment of 40/50.
- The CBCL 4–18 (Achenbach, 1991), filled in by Giuseppe's parents, gives pathological results in the internalising subscales: a) anxious/depressed (score 75%) and b) withdrawn/depressed (score 79%).

Diagnosis

The diagnosis is Obsessive-Compulsive Tic Disorder (OCTD, definition in Chapter 3).

The following P factors model (Dudley & Kuyken, 2006) is used in CBT to analyse clinical cases:

1   predisposing factors: born-with factors that increase the patient's risk to the problem.
2   precipitating factors: developmental events that have aggravated the problem.
3   perpetuating factors: elements maintaining the problem.
4   protective factors: patient's strengths for his psychological wellness, which may serve to enable recovery.

Predisposing factors

a   The subject has bilinear transmission for OC component, in this specific case the father has a severe OCTD. The parents' behavioural disturbance causes anxiety in Giuseppe as he feels loved and rewarded only as a result of excellent performances.

b   Giuseppe follows what's imposed by his family because of his personality traits, despite the developing personality of a 15-year-old boy. The subject could maintain in his adulthood an OC component because of the strictness of his cognitive and behavioural schemes, because of his low emotional insight and because of his OC positive genetics.

c   Giuseppe's social isolation, starting during primary school, doesn't allow him to enjoy school as a place of companionship and shared experiences, but merely as a place of commitment and productivity. Giuseppe's inflexible thinking and his behavioural stiffness make him very demanding of himself, developing very high educational objectives, difficult to maintain without a high level of stress and anxiety (Lazarus & Folkman, 1984).

Precipitating factors

a   Coughing tic onset is the main factor unsettling the patient: Giuseppe suddenly feels the weight of this disease, not knowing where it comes from and how to handle it. He chooses not to inform classmates and teachers about the problem and he therefore has to face it by himself, trying to cover it up, which requires huge physical, cognitive and emotional effort.

b   Starting high school leads to increasing duties, incrementing the level of stress.

c   Adolescence already comes with new social demands, requiring new skills to be developed (Erickson, 1950).

Perpetuating factors

a   Coughing is Giuseppe's most intense tic, and it is self-reproducing: it starts a vicious circle on a psychological and organic level, as it causes an airway rash. Clinicians agree on the interruption of trials of approaching school again if the cough lasts over 20 minutes. This choice also limits Giuseppe's attempts of approaching school again, already made unstable by the situation.

b   Giuseppe's avoidances represent another perpetuating factor. The main one is school absenteeism, resulting in school phobia and eventually school drop-out.

c   Parental expectations are too high, and they stayed as such if comparing them with when Giuseppe didn't show any difficulties in attending school. Parents are negatively reinforcing Giuseppe's efforts in studying or trying to attend school as they are used to awarding commitment only leading to brilliant successes.

d   Giuseppe doesn't care about his mates' text messages on his mobile phone when avoiding school. He is aware of his social isolation and he figures he would be bullied again by his mates if going back to school.

e   The teachers don't help with improving Giuseppe's condition, as they aim to maintain a high academic level, offering the same oral and written tests and pressuring him about his school attendance.

f   Giuseppe doesn't have any anchors as he doesn't have anyone to talk to about his complicated condition (Verdellen et al, 2011).

Alert!

Don't allow your child to skip school days because of a psychological disease! This may lead to developing more symptoms.

Protective factors

a   Giuseppe is gifted from an analytic point of view (left brain, cf. Wolman, 2012), and for this reason he has been a good candidate for cognitive behavioural therapy.

b   The activities he keeps attending to as hobbies are his resources: those activities allow him to spend some time outside his home, to finally be with his peers, and to be the winning leader of performances. Self-esteem takes great advantage from it as he is not able anymore to count on his scholastic success he has always been used to (Allen et al, 2018).

Psychotherapy pathway

The following programme is combined (as "add-on treatment": cf. Chapter 4) to medications, which modulate the neurotransmitters responsible of OCTD. Giuseppe attends weekly (and then increasingly less) sessions of Habit Reversal Training + other CBT techniques (cf. Chapter 4), first face to face, then taking part to online-based sessions, given the distance between the patient and the TS Centre (Dèttore et al, 2015). Sixty-five sessions had been attended overall.

At the same time, Parent Training is scheduled every 3 weeks, and then increasingly less (for a total of 26 sessions with parents). Meetings with school staff are scheduled on necessity (eight school meetings had been conducted).

Exposure and Response Prevention (ERP)

After psychoeducation sessions, Exposure and Response Prevention technique (cf. Chapter 4) is used, together with the diaphragmatic breathing technique (cf. Chapter 4) before facing each new task.

The hierarchy of Exposure and Response Prevention (Table 9.1) is first used on the less disturbing book for Giuseppe, his History book. The same technique can be applied to other books later on. Giuseppe is then asked to do something that involves school (e.g. going in front of his school and then coming back home), increasing slightly the level of stress to desensitise him to the anxiety stimulus, one step at the time. The boy has a specific homework assigned: to note the severity of the coughing symptom and of his satisfaction for overcoming each step.

Initially the patient, because of his anxiety, finds psychotherapy too complex. For this reason, he skips some steps; during sessions he would rather talk about his efforts to go to school when the request is only to try approaching the book again. Giuseppe goes back to attending school intermittently. The TS team congratulates with him reminding him to focus on the book and explaining the

Table 9.1 Hierarchy of Exposure and Response Prevention for the trigger "book". Giuseppe keeps track of his coughing severity and satisfaction levels, while approaching each task.

Approaching again the history book

	Date	Task	Coughing severity 0–10*	Satisfaction 0–10*
1	April, 1st week	Turning pages: 3 mins	2	4
2	April, 2nd week	Reading page numbers: 3 mins	1	4
3	April, 3rd week	Reading words from the bottom of the page to the top: 3 mins	2	5
4	April, 4th week	Reading a whole page from the bottom to the top: 5 mins	0	4
5	May, 1st week	Reading the index: 5 mins	3	4
6	May, 2nd week	Reading chapter titles: 5 mins	1	5
7	May, 3rd week	Reading half a page: mins needed	2	7
8	May, 4th week	Reading a page: mins needed	3	7
9	June, 1st week	Reading three pages: mins needed	2	7
10	June, 2nd week	Studying two pages: mins needed	0	8

* 10 meaning the highest and 0 the lowest

advantages of a gradual intervention that aims to get stable results, preventing relapses.

The way Giuseppe decides to go back to school is everything but gradual: he packs his school bag in an obsessive way and he prepares for all the classes, attending six hours of lessons, taking part in oral and written tests as every other student. Because of his flawless behaviour, after a school day, the anxiety levels became so high that Giuseppe is unable to go to school on the following days of the week. Giuseppe and the therapist dwell on his rushed approaching to school again, and they finally decide to desensitise approaching school with the same steps of approaching the history book (see Table 9.1), that has been overcome at the same time.

Given his first good results, Giuseppe's family pushes him to conclude his second high school year, trying for a private exam to be taken during the summer 2016. Clinicians don't agree with this parental proposal, they find it too risky (in case of failure) for such a psychologically weak subject. Parents believe it could give their son a chance and he agrees to try it. During the first three weeks the boy is able to study with low coughing attacks, then these symptoms increase, and he has to stop studying and consequently gives up on the exam, with intense feelings of disappointment.

Giuseppe and the therapist then try from where they stopped, working again on the Exposure and Response Prevention in approaching school. But his attempt to take the exams causes a relapse, even with an effect on homework, and they therefore go back to the ERP focusing on books. When this ERP is overcome, the technique can finally be applied to school attendance.

Cognitive diary and ABC technique

These CBT techniques (cf. Chapter 4; see Table 9.2) have been aiming to restore Giuseppe's psychological wellness within his peer relationships. Once Giuseppe realises his typical cognitive biases (e.g. inflexible thinking), he can self-monitor through his daily cognitive diary, looking for new and more functional options of thinking (Dèttore, 2003).

The psychological intervention involves Giuseppe, his parents and teachers, who are invited to modify their attitude towards the boy's school performances. This has been a key point of the therapy and, most of all, for finding once more the authentic "unconditional positive regard" (Rogers, 1995) given to Giuseppe by his role model adults, despite his poor results in trying to attend school. The renowned psychotherapist Rogers, in his Person-Centred approach, talks about unconditional love as an attitude of valuing each other, even knowing there are failings.

Table 9.2 ABC example in Giuseppe's cognitive diary. Thoughts are reported between brackets. Emotion level is 0 to a maximum of 10.

A (antecedents)	B (problem)	C (consequences)	Reflections & alternatives
11th November Home alone "All my friends smoke"	"All my friends are a disaster" Sadness 8/10	"I am lonely, and noone is like me" Loneliness 8.5/10	In my thoughts I made a generalisation (word "everyone") and a catastrophisation (word "disaster"): Not everyone smokes and it's not a reason good enough to think they are a disaster, they have other qualities. They are my friends because there is something in them that I like. This implies I am not lonely. Tomorrow I will try to hang out with them and I will see how it goes.

In practice, the parents are advised on how to positively reinforce Giuseppe's even slight efforts in approaching homework and school, and they are asked to quit negative reinforcements and their dysfunctional ignoring the boy (e.g. at the beginning they aren't reinforcing his small trials of approaching the book). Moreover, the parents are explained to that this is a disorder that needs a gradual therapeutic program. Therefore, it is counter-productive to follow Giuseppe's request to move to the next step of ERP more quickly than agreed with the therapist. The parents are also invited to be more affectionate, with homework such as a daily "family hug" (Bevilacqua & Dattilio, 2010) at a pre-set time, thus to increase the manifestation of positive emotions in a low-Expressed-Emotion family (Brown & Rutter, 1966).

Teachers are advised to gently welcome the boy in class, and not to ask for homework and not to impose oral or written class tests, despite Giuseppe needing marks so as to avoid failing a year, and even if it is fundamental for the teachers themselves. The therapist shares with the teachers the ERP schedule for a gradual approach to school, and understanding the rationale they decide to follow it, with the approval of the school principal. In agreement with Giuseppe and his family, a meeting between the student's class, the student himself and his clinicians is also arranged in order to inform his schoolmates about main syndrome's features and how they can behave to best support him.

Alert!

School staff should focus on non-performance topics in the case of students with school-related disorders.

Outcome

Medical treatment and psychological interventions, namely HRT, Parent Training and school meetings, improved Giuseppe's condition.

During the winter of 2016–2017, his school attendance peaked at 40%, but this was not sustained over a longer period. From January to March 2017, Giuseppe's attendance was 20%; he later completed all ERP phases, returning to a full attendance in his third year of high school.

With regards to mood, the boy started, step by step, to discuss his strict way of thinking and to recognise his biases, thanks to psychoeducation and CBT techniques such as the cognitive diary and the ABC. He became open to new points of view as, conscious of his own discomfort, he motivated himself to do his best to recover.

Through restructuring his thoughts and changing his behaviours, OCTD issues gradually improved. As a consequence, the boy could interrupt his medical treatment. Giuseppe started to develop friendships within his athletics group, among schoolmates and in the neighbourhood, and he even experienced his first romance. Now Giuseppe is 17, he attends school regularly, he has been in a genuine sentimental relationship for a month and he knows how important it is to be part of a group and to have a social life. He promises himself he won't have a setback. In the future, he would love to study Physics at university. The psychotherapy pathway ended after three years.

Retest and follow-up

When the treatment was concluded (May 2018), a retest was proposed to Giuseppe and his parents. The same three scales filled out in baseline gave the following results:

- CY-BOCS value: 7/40, thus indicating absence of OC component.
- YGTSS value: 20% with 5/50 of Social Impairment, which means tics being mild and well-accepted.
- CBCL 4-18 (2 internalising subscales) values: anxious/depressed (score 50%), withdrawn/depressed (score 52%), i.e. absence of anxiety or depression symptoms.

Follow-up meetings, aiming to prevent possible relapses, were scheduled after two weeks, then after three weeks, and the final one after one month.

Therapeutic relationship

Giuseppe interacted with his psychotherapist in a fluctuating manner, considering his mood symptomatology: sometimes equipped with confidence and having a good insight on the pathology, other times being reluctant and underestimating the clinician, almost testing her. This attitude of being oppositional was part of his spectrum, but the therapist herself affirmed she frequently needed to make an effort to carry on the session in an empathic way. Giuseppe often discussed the expertise of his psychotherapist (e.g. the efficacy of the techniques she was offering him), implying her level of professionalism may have not been up to standard. This had an influence on the patient's motivation to accurately do homework. Nevertheless, during the course of treatment, the sufferer's and caregivers' compliance increased, facilitating the therapeutic management overall.

Conclusions

Giuseppe's case underlines the efficacy of combining ad hoc psychotherapeutic intervention and medical treatment in OCTD patients. The two therapies are considered *combinable* and *variable* (or an add-on treatment) during the cure pathway in order to optimise that specific patient's biopsychosocial wellness. The involvement of caregivers, i.e. Giuseppe's family and school, facilitated an improvement in Social Impairment. Readers should bear in mind that even if Social Impairment is the reason motivating a treatment in TS, the syndrome has an organic nature.

References

Achenbach T. 1991. *Manual for the Child Behavior Checklist for Ages 4–18 (CBCL 4-18)*. Burlington, VT, USA: University Associate on Psychiatry.

Allen CW, Diamond-Myrsten S, & Rollins LK. 2018. School Absenteeism in Children and Adolescents. Vol *98*(12). *American Family Physician*, 738–744.

Bevilacqua LJ & Dattilio FM. 2010. *Family Therapy Homework Planner, second edition*. Hoboken, NJ, USA: John Wiley and Sons, 175.

Brown GW & Rutter M. 1966. The measurement of family activities and relationships: A methodological study. Vol *19*. *Human Relations*, 741–763.

Dell'Osso B, Marazziti D, Albert U, Pallanti S, Gambini O, Tundo A, . . . , & Porta M. 2017. Parsing the phenotype of obsessive-compulsive tic disorder (OCTD): A multidisciplinary consensus. Vol *21*(2). *International Journal of Psychiatry in Clinical Practice*, 156–159.

Dèttore D. 2003. *Il disturbo ossessivo-compulsivo: Caratteristiche cliniche e tecniche di intervento*. Milano, IT, EU: McGraw-Hill, 213–224.

Dèttore D, Pozza A, & Andersson G. 2015. Efficacy of technology-delivered cognitive behavioural therapy for OCD versus control conditions, and in comparison with therapist-administered CBT: Meta-analysis of randomized controlled trials. Vol *44*(3). *Cognitive Behavior Therapy*, 190–211.

Dudley R & Kuyken W. 2006. Formulation in Cognitive Behavioural Therapy. In: Johnstone L & Dallos R, eds. *Formulation in Psychology and Psychotherapy*. New York, NY, USA: Routledge, 17–46.

Erickson H. 1950. Childhood and Society. New York, NY, USA: W.W. Norton & Co, 275–284.

Gava I, Barbui C, Aguglia E, Carlino D, Churchill R, De Vanna M, & McGuire HF. 2007. Psychological treatments versus treatment as usual for obsessive compulsive disorder (OCD). Vol *2*. *Cochrane Database of Systematic Reviews*. CD005333.

Lazarus RS & Folkman S. 1984. *Stress, Appraisal and Coping*. New York, NY, USA: Springer Publishing Company, 226–257.

Leckman JF, Riddle MA, Hardin MT, Ort SI, Swartz KL, Stevenson J, & Cohen DJ. 1989. The Yale Global Tic Severity Scale: Initial testing of a clinician-rated scale of severity. Vol *28*. *Journal of the American Academy of Child & Adolescent Psychiatry*, 566–573.

Leckman JF. 2003. Phenomenology of tics and natural history of tic disorders. Vol 25(1). *Brain Development*, 24–28. Review.

Pozza A, Giaquinta N, & Dèttore D. 2015. The contribution of alexithymia to obsessive-compulsive disorder symptoms dimensions: An investigation in a large community sample in Italy. *Psychiatry Journal*. 707850. doi: 10.1155/2015/707850.

Robertson MM, Eapen V, Singer HS, Martino D, Scharf JM, & Paschou P, . . . , & Leckman JF. 2017. Gilles de la Tourette syndrome. Vol 3. *Nature Reviews Disease Primers*, 16097. doi: 10.1038/nrdp.2016.97.

Rogers C. 1995. *On Becoming a Person: A Therapist's View of Psychotherapy*. Boston, MA, USA: Houghton Mifflin Harcourt, 314–328.

Scahill L, Riddle MA, McSwiggin-Hardin M, Ort SI, King RA, Goodman WK, . . . , & Leckman JF. 1997. Children's Yale-Brown Obsessive Compulsive Scale: reliability and validity. Vol 36(6). *Journal of the American Academy of Child & Adolescent Psychiatry*, 844–852.

Verdellen C, van de Griendt J, Hartmann A, Murphy T, & ESSTS Guidelines Group. 2011. European clinical guidelines for Tourette syndrome and other tic disorders. Part III: Behavioural and psychosocial interventions. Vol 20(4). *European Child & Adolescent Psychiatry*, 197–207.

Wolman D. 2012. The split brain: A tale of two halves. Vol 483(7389). *Nature*, 260–263.

Glossary

ABC analysis CBT technique; the patient is asked to analyse the situation describing feelings, thoughts and behaviours of a problematic episode. 'ABC' refers to the different chronological moments of the episode. The patient is then asked to make some reflections on the episode, and to give alternatives in thinking or behaviour.

anamnesis A preliminary case history of a patient.

attention-deficit/hyperactivity disorder (ADHD) Neuro-developmental disorder including a deficiency of attention and/or motor restlessness, excessive need for activity and high impulsivity.

autism spectrum disorder A broad range of neurodevelopmental disorders, characterised by deficits in social skills (communication and interaction), and other cognitive-behavioural symptoms. The broad range varies depending on symptoms, skills and levels of impairment.

botulinum toxin Neurotoxin used in medicine to treat different conditions, such as disorders characterised by overactive muscles.

central nervous system (CNS) Part of the nervous system, together with the peripheral nervous system. It is divided between the brain and spinal cord. It is made of neurons and tissue connecting neurons.

cerebellum One of the structures of the nervous system. It is responsible for learning and coordination of complex movements (e.g. walking).

chorea Neurological disorder characterised by abrupt involuntary movements. The term derives from the Greek word "dance".

clinical scales Standardised tests used in medicine to assess patients' pathologies.

clonic tic   Quick, snap tics (e.g. blinking).

Cognitive Behavioural Therapy (CBT)   Evidence-based psycho-therapy; mainly structured by sessions with a therapist. The aim of CBT is to work with the patient on changing dysfunctional thoughts and behavioural patterns, to have a positive effect on their emotional regulation.

(cognitive-behavioural) diary   CBT technique used to self-monitor dysfunctional cognitive, behavioural and emotional symptoms.

compliance   Patients' and caregivers' adherence to clinicians' prescriptions during the diagnostic-therapeutic pathway.

connectivity   Patterns of links between distinct units in a nervous system. Brain connectivity is thus crucial to elucidating how neurons and neural networks process information.

coprolalia   Tic consisting of the repetition of obscene word/s or sentences out of context.

copropraxia   Tic consisting of the repetition of obscene movements out of context.

cortex   Part of the brain regulating the "superior activities" (e.g. attention, awareness and thought).

cranial nerves   Nerves emerging from the brain and belonging to the peripheral nervous system.

Deep Brain Stimulation (DBS)   Neurosurgical procedure con-sisting of the implanting two electrodes to stimulate a patient's specific brain nuclei.

dyscalculia   Specific learning disability in math, such as difficulty in performing arithmetical calculations.

dysgraphia   Specific learning disorder that affects written expres-sion, mostly handwriting but also coherence.

dyslexia   Specific learning disorder causing difficulties mostly with reading, spelling and writing.

dystonic tic   tic characterised by the patient miming dysfunc-tional postures (e.g. teeth grinding). It is slower than clonic tics.

echolalia   Tic characterised by the repetition of someone else's word/s. It must be out of context.

echopraxia   Tic characterised by the repetition of someone else's movements. It must be out of context.

ecophenomena   Tics' category including echolalia and echopraxia (see definitions in this glossary).

etiopathology   Study of the causes of pathologies.

Exposure and Response Prevention (ERP)   CBT technique consisting in the gradual exposure of the patient to the anxious stimulus, preventing the usual symptoms (anxiety, nervousness, etc.), thanks to the use of other techniques such as the dia-phragmatic breathing.

extrapyramidal system Part of the motor system network producing involuntary movements. It includes basal ganglia, and plays a key role in tics' production.

functional magnetic resonance imaging Technique for measuring brain activity by detecting changes associated with blood flow. This technique is also used for the study of connectivity and plasticity (see definitions in the glossary).

gene Basic physical and functional unit of heredity for living beings. The branch of biology concerned with the study of genes is genetics.

Habit Reversal Training (HRT) CBT method for Tourette syndrome patients. The training mainly promotes the symptoms' awareness, and an alternative movement, i.e. "a new habit" in contrast with a target tic, together with the use of other CBT techniques.

hypothalamus Small region of the brain, located under the thalamus. It regulates the sense of appetite, body temperature, sleep-wake cycle and other essential functions.

impulse control disorder Disorder characterized by impulsivity, i.e. failure to resist an urge or impulse. One type of impulse control disorder is kleptomania (i.e. pathological stealing).

learning disorder Neurological condition causing disabilities processing information. It can interfere with learning basic skills such as reading, writing and/or maths.

limbic system System made of central nervous system's interacting structures. The latter are responsible for actions' related emotions and memories, influencing the "how/when" of doing something. The limbic system regulates impulses and behaviours linked to several self-conservative mechanisms, such as nutrition.

malignant tic Painful tics (e.g. a frequent neck roll tic causing pain).

microglia Cells located in the brain and in the spinal cord with the role of immune protectors.

mirror neurons A group of neurons that fires both when a person (or animal) acts and when the person (or animal) observes, in a sort of mirroring, the same action performed by another person (or animal).

neurobehavioural disease Cognitive, behavioural and emotional disorders associated with damage or dysfunction in the central nervous system.

neuroleptic   Class of drugs used to treat and manage symptoms of many neuropsychiatric disorders.

neuron   Fundamental unit of the nervous system; it is an electrically excitable cell holding information and communicating with other cells.

neurotransmitter   Substances, whose release connects neurons. Serotonin is an example of a neurotransmitter, modulating mood and other processes.

Non-Obscene Socially Inappropriate behaviours (NOSI)   Behavioural symptom, characterised by inappropriate behaviours or tics (e.g. shouting out "bomb" in an airport).

OC component   The term used in the Manual for Obsessive-Compulsive Behaviour, Obsessive-Compulsive Disorder and Obsessive-Compulsive Symptoms. It is a disorder characterised by obsessions (intrusive, undesired repetitive ideas, or images for a specific object, which can be a living being or inanimate) and compulsions (repetitive undesired actions or thoughts, used by the patient to block obsessions). See details in Chapter 3.

oppositional defiant disorder   Behavioural disorder including rage/irritable mood, controversial behaviour or revenge.

palilalia   Tic characterised by the repetition of one's own utterance. It must be out of context.

Paediatric Autoimmune Neuropsychiatric Disorders Associated with group A beta-haemolytic Streptococcal Infections (PANDAS)   Childhood acute-onset spectrum composed by various TS-like symptoms (e.g. handwriting tics). Symptoms may arise after streptococcal infections, and they occur in the form of severe attacks.

Parent Training   CBT training sessions aiming to help the parents of a patient to manage their child's specific disease.

peripheral nervous system (PNS)   Part of the nervous system, together with the central nervous system. Made of nerves, it is located outside the brain and the spinal cord. Its main function is exchanging information between the central nervous system and the rest of the body.

personality disorder   Psychiatric disorder characterised by patients thinking, feeling, behaving or relating to others very differently when compared with a healthy person. There are several different types of personality disorder; an example is the dependent personality disorder (characterised by pervasive need to be taken care of that leads to submissive behaviour and other symptoms).

plasticity The brain's ability to change and adapt to experience.

premonitory urge Physical/psychological urgency, which signals the tic arrival.

psychogenic tic Tic caused by a psychological disease.

psychological disease Cognitive or behavioural pattern causing significant distress or impairment of personal functioning.

Quality of Life (QoL) Level of well-being (regarding health, family, education, employment, safety, wealth, etc.) experienced by an individual or group.

refractory Disease that resists a specific treatment.

school phobia Anxiety disorder characterised by the specific phobia/fear/preoccupation for the school context. School's absenteeism is the typical behaviour of the patient suffering from this disorder.

Self-Injurious Behaviour (SIB) Behavioural symptom, characterised by self-harm (e.g. hit your own knee against a table) without an intention of death.

social anxiety Disorder characterised by intense anxiety or fear of being judged, negatively evaluated or rejected in a social or performance situation. It leads to negative thoughts and feelings of inadequacy, inferiority, embarrassment, humiliation and depression, and to behaviours such as avoiding specific social contexts.

Social Impairment Social disease (e.g. isolation) of an individual or group, given by pathologies or other conditions.

Selective Serotonin Reuptake Inhibitors (SSRIs) A class of antidepressant drugs, including Sertraline.

stuttering Speech disorder characterised by involuntary disruptions such as repetitions of sounds/syllables/words, or prolongation of sounds, or interruptions of speech. It has the same neurological basis as tics.

thalamus Region located in the middle of the brain. It is a "transit and sorting station" for a) sensory, b) motor and c) behavioural information.

tic(s) Repetitive, nonrhythmic and purposeless movement(s). They may be motor tics (e.g. blinking) or sound tics (e.g. coughing).

token economy   CBT technique in which tokens are won/lost when the child behaves correctly/incorrectly. A sum of tokens for a specific time period is rewarded with a prize.

tonic tic   Tic characterised by a progressive muscular contraction (e.g. arm stretching). It is slower than dystonic tics.

Tourette syndrome (TS)   Neurodevelopmental disease characterised by more than a motor tic and at least a sound tic. Onset is before age 18. Other features of TS are detailed in Chapter 3.

trichotillomania   Psychological disorder, characterised by the urge to pull out one's hair.

Postscript

In conclusion, the authors would like to donate a humble teaching to readers, both experts and caregivers. If we go back more than 2,200 years, the Rosetta Stone can help us in this task (Figure 10.1). It was discovered in 1799 by a French soldier during the Napoleonic campaign in Egypt. It reports a decree, written in hieroglyphic script, demotic script and ancient Greek. The comparison between the three languages made possible the translation of the previously unknown hieroglyphic script, opening a window into Egyptian history. In the same way, the comparison between Tourette syndrome symptoms and other pathologies, has clarified previously unknown symptoms (Figure 10.1).

Research in many medical areas, not only in neurology or psychiatry, has led to the study of ADHD and OC component. Today they might no longer be considered as separate patterns from tics, but as part of the uniqueness of Tourette syndrome. The TS motor-sensory hyperarousal, and the relationship between TS and the microglia's dysfunction, help understanding the syndrome as having a neurological base. For this reason, Tourette syndrome patients cannot benefit from psychoanalytic or other traditional psychological interventions! Neurotransmitters need to be resettled through medication or cognitive exercises, but in mild cases, no intervention is needed. For those fortunate to work with people having Tourette syndrome, they should recognise it is an extraordinary experience. Many TS sufferers are gifted with a "joy of living", "feel like doing" attitude and creativity. These features can be a source of enthusiasm or frustration to clinicians, according to the time of syndrome's evolution and to positive or negative therapeutic results. Families of TS patients usually actively participate

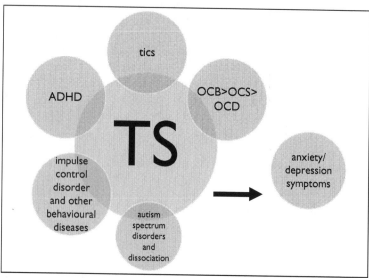

Figure 10.1 Rosetta Stone and TS spectrum: identification of new languages (top) and symptoms (bottom).

Credit: Cecilia Spalletti.

during the diagnostic-therapeutic pathway, sometimes with their own difficulties. Experts are trained to prevent these difficulties and intervene when necessary. Teamwork is mandatory as the sufferer needs to feel at the centre of a coworking group. TS specialists could not work separately as one would impinge upon the other. Intervention should be patient-oriented, and all clinicians and caregivers should be "at the patient's service", by educating, and curing with care. A *fortiori*, when the affected is a child, proper management guarantees a better future Quality of Life.

Questionnaire

Please answer the following questions about the information you read in the book. Only one answer is correct. This can help you define your understanding of Tourette symdrome (TS).

1 Tourette syndrome is a:

    a   neurological disease
    b   psychological disease
    c   neurodevelopmental disease with behavioural implications

2 The main skill of a TS patient is:

    a   creativity
    b   computer ability
    c   a specific talent with building blocks

3 Stakeholders of a TS child are:

    a   irrelevant. He has to be self-efficient
    b   family, school staff and a TS team of clinicians
    c   grandparents and special needs teachers

4 Why does the law need special attention in the Tourette's world?

    a   patients can be involved in legal issues
    b   clinicians can be involved in legal issues
    c   patients, families and clinicians can be involved in legal issues

5 Who was the first TS sufferer?

    a   Marquise De Dampierre
    b   Charcot
    c   Georges Albert Édouard Brutus Gilles de la Tourette

6 Giuseppe (in Chapter 9) was suffering from:

   a   Tourette syndrome
   b   a subtype of TS with predominant OC component
   c   tics, coughing and OC component

7 In a case of school phobia, a parent should:

   a   make sure the child goes to school
   b   allow the child to stay home
   c   ask for a psychological consultation. Usually the best attitude is to send the child to school

8 When in front of tics, a family should:

   a   ignore tics
   b   ask the child the reason of his manifestations
   c   smile at the child

9 It is advised to base hobbies on:

   a   TS parents' preferences
   b   the TS child's interests and passions
   c   the socialisation of the TS sufferer

10 Therapies in TS:

   a   can be associated
   b   are pharmacological
   c   are psychological

Correct answers: 1c, 2a, 3b, 4c, 5a, 6b, 7c, 8a, 9b, 10a.

Contributors

Alberto Riccardo Bona, M.D. Neurosurgery – Functional Neurosurgery, Galeazzi Clinical and Research Hospital of Milan

Matteo Briguglio, M.Sc. Food and Nutrition – Tourette Syndrome Centre, Galeazzi Clinical and Research Hospital of Milan

Donatella Comasini, M.Sc. Psychology – Associazione Italiana Sindrome Tourette

Davide Dèttore, Professor Psychology – University of Florence

Roberta Galentino, M.Sc. Psychology – Tourette Syndrome Centre, Galeazzi Clinical and Research Hospital of Milan

Selenia Greco, M.Sc. Psychology, 2nd lev. Masters – Associazione Italiana Sindrome Tourette

Thomas Spalletti, B.Sc. Psychology – University of Turin

Index